REWIRING PAIN:

A new way to reclaim your life

||||||||||||||||||||||||||||||||||||||||||||||||||||||||||||||||||||||||||||||||||||||||||||||||||||||||||||||||||||||||||||||||||||||||

Dr Lisa Chaffey

(ClinScD)

Published in Australia in 2019

By Lisa Chaffey
www.lisachaffey.com.au

 A catalogue record for this
book is available from the
NATIONAL
LIBRARY National Library of Australia
OF AUSTRALIA

Chaffey, Lisa

Rewiring pain. The new way to reclaim your life / Lisa
Chaffey

ISBN: 978 0 6485010 0 8 (pbk)
ISBN: 978 0 6485010 1 5 (ebook)

For all who stood by me when the going got tough. And for all of you who are currently going through similar tough times.

This book is about my experience of managing chronic pain. The advice contained is of a general nature only. Please seek medical advice for issues that arise.

About the author

Lisa has a Doctorate in Clinical Science from La Trobe University, Melbourne. She is an occupational therapist, academic and researcher.

Before developing chronic pain, Lisa was a member of the Australian women's wheelchair basketball team. She has a silver medal from the Athens Paralympics (2004), and two bronze medals from the 1994 and 2002 World championships.

To read more about Lisa, visit her website: www.lisachaffey.com.au

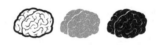

Contents

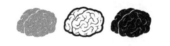

Introduction

Chronic pain is awful. There is no other way of saying it. It's like carrying a sack of potatoes. A sack that you can never put down, no matter how weary you become. No matter how busy your life. No matter how much that sack gets in the way. It doesn't even matter how heavy the sack is; it's tiring simply because it's always there.

That is, until now. Advances in medical imaging technology has opened up a whole new world of knowledge about the brain. Research on neuroplasticity (how the brain changes itself) has opened up. Science can now see what happens in the brain for a person in pain.

This book introduces you to simple, but effective methods to reduce chronic pain. Using the scientific discoveries from neuroplasticity research, everyday activities and habits are turned into pain competitors. This book provides a step-by-step guide to help you rewire your brain, create your own path out of pain and reclaim your life.

Obviously, there needs to be a good reason why someone would spend hours, weeks, months, and years of their life writing a book. For me, this book arose from my own battle with chronic pain. It was a battle that started out of the blue. It was a battle that only ended after I found a way to combine current research on brain plasticity and activities from occupational therapy to rewire pain processes in my brain.

I have spent a lifetime dealing with frequent pain, normally lasting a day or two. I was born with a rare spinal disability, resulting in a shortened torso and paralysed legs. Half of the bones in my spine are missing, so I frequently have acute pain at the base of my spine. Fortunately, I can minimise the chance of getting pain if I am careful. And by 'careful', I mean 'wrapping myself in cotton wool'. However, I choose to live a full and active life and to deal with any pain as it arises. But at the end of 2013, something else happened that pushed my acute pain to chronic pain, and the wind was knocked out of my sails.

I went searching for a way to manage my pain and still live my life. I am an occupational therapists and post-doctoral research fellow, so naturally I delved into research publications and ended up in the worlds of occupational therapy theory, neuroscience and behaviour. I spent months researching and reading about the mechanisms of acute pain, and how that slowly sneaks into the lifestyle and habits of chronic pain. The more I understood what was happening, the less fearful I was.

And then, the sudden light bulb went off as I began to read research about how pain changes patterns and pathways in the brain, and how it is possible to weaken those pain pathways and rewire your brain. I combined this idea about the brain making new connections and pathways with ideas from my occupational therapy training about activities, habits and daily routines.

Based on the research and my occupational therapy training, I started to use every day activities to rewire the pain processes in my brain. But more than that, I could personalise the activities, changing them according to my pain levels in each day/hour. Using these strategies, I reduced my pain over several months to just a niggle here and there.

Let me start by telling you my story. Then, I will lead

you through the research that I found and show you how I used my brain to defeat pain.

My story

I was dreading the long flight home from Bangkok to Melbourne. I looked around the gate lounge and the scene in front of me was of bored teenagers, crying toddlers, and frazzled parents. The next eight hours was going to be uncomfortable, noisy, and seem like an eternity. Tired from my week of work in Bangkok, I knew that I needed to spend the next three days marking 140 or so assignments that were waiting in my pigeonhole at the medical school back home. So, I made a choice. A choice that seemed inconsequential at the time, but a choice that shaped the next two years of my life.

That choice? I took a sleeping tablet.

To understand how that sleeping tablet led to two years of chronic pain, I need to take you back to the day I was born, 44 years earlier.

It was 8am on a Saturday in a scorching Australian summer when I came into the world. I was tiny, and yet I managed to cause quite a commotion in the labour ward. Something was wrong. I had long, dark eyelashes, cute dimples, and a powerful set of lungs, but I had only half my vertebra, or back bone. My legs were paralysed and twisted, and my torso was half the length that it should have been. The doctors figured that my internal organs were being squashed. The priest was called for. I wasn't meant to stick around for very long. Luckily, I was stubborn.

Being stubborn came in handy in my childhood. It meant that I persisted until I became good at using my callipers and crutches, and then my wheelchair. The area that should have been the base of my spine (if I had the right number of vertebrae) ached at the end of most days, but the pain was usually gone by morning. I spent a lot of time in hospital, with more than my fair share of surgery. But, despite all that pain, I remember a fun and active childhood.

The other neighbourhood kids and I adapted games to integrate disability long before it was cool. I learnt to read when I was three, and the special school for kids with disabilities was no longer enough for me. I was only the second child in my city to be integrated into a mainstream school, once again, before it was cool. Then, I went to university and trained as an occupational therapist. Of course, I didn't do any of this alone. I had friends, parents and an older brother who encouraged, challenged and supported me.

My family and friends supported me once again as they cheered on the Australian women's wheelchair basketball team, The Gliders, when we won a Silver medal at the 2004 Athens Paralympics. I was one of the shortest players in the world, but I was known for my stubbornness on the court. One of my favourite descriptions of my game came from the brief player biographies in the 2003 National Women's Wheelchair Basketball League program: 'Lisa Chaffey (#6): Short in stature, but tough as nails'.

And I was tough ... until an elbow injury ended my playing career at the first national training camp after Athens, as we started our campaign for the 2008 Beijing Paralympics.

Just like that, my sporting career was over.

But I was not quite ready to let go of the sport I loved, so I trained as a basketball technical official – a classifier. It was my job to classify a player's level of disability based on their body function and movements when playing the game that I so desperately wanted to play myself. Surprisingly though, I loved classifying almost as much as I loved playing, and I set about classifying at national and international wheelchair basketball events.

Quitting basketball forced me to think about the 'what next', the 'plan B'. I figured that I would have a lot of free time after stopping elite level competition, so the day after I retired from basketball, I enrolled in a clinical doctorate in occupational therapy. I spent six years examining the use of intuition in clinical practice. Early on in that process, a colleague gave me an important piece of advice. She said that you don't necessarily have to be smart to complete a doctorate, but you do have to be persistent. Persistent/stubborn ... same thing.

I worked in clinical occupational therapy for a few years and then I moved into research and academia, which I loved. I was in a privileged position of teaching and conducting research in health. I loved the opportunity to explore areas of interest, to delve into a subject and to bring theories from dry academic articles into everyday practice.

And so, flying home on the red-eye from Thailand, after being a classifier at the Asia Oceania Wheelchair Basketball Championships, getting ready to mark 140 student assignments, I had to make a choice: jet lag or a sleeping tablet. In hindsight, I made the wrong decision, one that would cause chronic pain, but we wouldn't link that choice to my pain for another year.

The beginning of my chronic pain journey began, like many do, with what I thought was a simple acute illness. On the first day back at work, marking those 140 assignments at my desk, a sudden hideous pain gripped my entire abdomen. The kind of pain that demanded attention. The only way to describe it is to say that electric shocks sparked all over my torso and I felt like I had a rock sitting in my abdomen. I had cramps, or I really should say, one vice-like grip of a cramp. I was nauseous and I was flushed.

The pain was relentless, but I thought it was probably just a stomach bug that I picked up in Thailand, so I took a coffee break to catch my breath. Then I tried to concentrate and finish marking those assignments. After all, I was 'tough as nails'.

Two days later, (two days of still trying to work) when this pattern persisted and I had not improved, my 'toughness' deserted me. My colleague bundled me into the car and drove to the nearest hospital emergency department. I never did finish marking those assignments.

That trip to hospital was the beginning of a pain journey that might be similar to yours. The emergency doctors found nothing specific to account for my pain. They too thought it might have been a stomach bug from Thailand. They sent me away with a prescription for painkillers and advice to follow-up with a gastrointestinal specialist if the pain continued.

Sure enough, the pain persisted. I met with the specialist at his earliest available appointment, three long weeks later. He also could not pinpoint the precise cause of pain, so ordered a battery of tests. Those tests came back clear, so he ordered a new batch of different tests. I spent Christmas Eve 2013 drinking radioactive fluid and lying on the CT scan bed. Yet, after all those tests, he found no cause for my pain.

For the next 12 months, my search for answers went something like this:

1. A visit to an interested doctor. Typically, the doctor was more interested in my rare spinal disability, and they couldn't see an obvious cause for my belly pain.

2. A range of medical tests would be ordered, all of which meant time off work, extra expenses and sometimes, hospital stays.

3. A trial of medication or dietary modification would be suggested.

4. Nothing would be found. My pain did not change.

5. A referral was made to another specialist who was knowledgeable about a different body part, and who suspected a new cause of my pain.

6. Return to step 1.

In the meantime, my pain had morphed from acute to chronic without me noticing that slide. Suddenly, it consumed every part of my daily life.

I had graduated to opioid-based medication, but my pain did not respond to that at all. The best I could hope for was that the medication would send me to sleep and the pain would have lessened by the time I awoke. I was also one of the unlucky few who experienced an opioid hangover in the morning, doubling the difficulties of living a life.

Unsurprisingly, slowly but surely, my world shrunk.

My social life was restricted to within a 200-metre radius of my couch, except on special occasions, and even then, I probably wouldn't make it. If I did make it to the event or party, I was reduced to wearing my 'good tracksuit pants' because anything more restrictive caused pain. My friends became experts at creating their own back-up plans because of the frequency with which I had to cancel at the last minute.

My career suffered too. I went to work but I struggled to sit at the computer for an entire day. Two months after the pain began, I interviewed for the permanent role of the casual job in the medical school I had been doing for six months, (the one with the 140 assignments that needed marking). The interview was conducted one week after I had exploratory surgery. Well, I don't remember much of the interview, but I know that despite preparing my answers in advance, I could not tell the panel anything about my skills. I was so consumed with managing my pain and getting by that I had nothing extra to offer. The bottom line was I just couldn't do it.

'I just couldn't do it' became a constant threat to the way I wanted to live my life, as I tried desperately to cling to my normality. I was angry because I was beginning to lose everything I had worked for, and I was fearful of the future.

Luckily, I was stubborn.

When the doctors could not solve my problem, I started using my research skills and resources to search for my own answers. I spent 12 long months trying anything that might give me some relief. My dietary strategies included: gluten-free, sugar-free, meat-free, alcohol-free, and fibre-free diets. Let me tell you, after a while those diets become fun-free and social life-free. I tried relaxation tapes and mindfulness meditation, and I slept better, but the pain did not change. But my biggest strategy at that time was just simply trying to cling to normality and to live my everyday life. Keeping that goal was what solved the mystery of the source of my pain, and then created the challenge to stop it.

It was December 3, 2014: almost a year to the day that the pain had begun. Part of the normality I wanted to cling to was attending the Christmas lunch of the Australian women's wheelchair basketball team. At an international tournament, like the Paralympic games, you need to be able to look down the bench and see the 11 other people you would go into battle with, because that is exactly what you are doing. You battle hard, sometimes winning, sometimes losing, but you always fight together. Those women from the Australian wheelchair basketball team were, and remain, the toughest people I know. Sure, I was once 'tough as nails' but now I was 'weak as a kitten', and I needed to tap into their collective strength.

Going to the lunch meant flying interstate and taking a two-hour train ride, but it was always worth it. In fact, at the end of such a horrible year, it was essential to me and my state of mind.

The day after the lunch, I was staying at a teammate's house, reading a book she had helped launch about pain in spinal cord injuries. Reading the book about common causes of pain for people with spinal cord injury, sitting in the sunshine beside the Brisbane Waters in Woy Woy, suddenly, the penny dropped.

My belly was not the problem. My spine was the culprit, or more specifically, my spinal nerves. Sitting on that plane from Thailand in 2013, not moving for eight hours because I had taken a sleeping pill, had annoyed a nerve in my 'creatively-arranged' spinal cord. My nerve was stuck in a perpetual feedback loop, malfunctioning and sending the wrong message to my brain that something drastic was happening in my abdomen. That is, I could feel pain, but there was no abdominal cause. It was neuropathic pain, pain caused by the wrong message from nerves.

Of course, it was neuropathic pain. The picture fitted perfectly: pain like electricity, burning, not responding to traditional pain medication, not even opioids. Now I knew what it was, all the fear disappeared. Pain was now only a nerve sensation, not scary. And I was no longer fearful that I was secretly dying.

When I got back to my office at the university the following week, I conducted a quick and dirty literature review, and visited my doctor with a shopping list of preferred drugs. I thought I would be fine, and everything would go back to normal, and yet ...

The relief of finally having a diagnosis was short lived in that first conversation with my doctor. He told me that neuropathic pain was typically resistant to medication and it may not respond at all. For me, that meant the burning electric shocks travelling through my belly were likely to be present for many more years to come.

I was lucky enough that one of the medications I was prescribed took the edge off my pain. The pain occurred less often, was less intense, and did not seem to last as long as it had before the medication. However, it was still there, just like a perpetual sack of potatoes. And I was also experiencing some weird side effects, such as unbearable fatigue and dreams that were like an episode of 'CSI'. In short, I was a little bit better but certainly not functioning the way I would like in my daily life. After four months, I made the decision to stop taking that medication.

Just as I feared, the pain returned.

Spending my whole life in a wheelchair, I'm adept at finding other ways to do things. So, when it was clear that the standard treatment for pain management was not going to make much of a difference for me, I decided to tackle this pain like I tackled playing hide and seek in the schoolyard or playing good offence on a basketball court. I decided to out-think the obstacles and find another way.

Using my research skills, I went back to the science and health literature to look at new and emerging ideas. And then ... I made a discovery. I stumbled on a Ted talk by Lorimer Mosely, a professor and physiotherapist from South Australia who researches chronic pain and the world of neuroscience. His talk and his books opened my eyes about using the brain to defeat chronic pain.

From that initial discovery, I branched out to other books such as Norman Doidge's, *The brain's way of healing*[1], and Michael Moskowitz's, *Neuroplastic*

---

1   Doidge, N. (2016). *The Brain's Way of Healing: remarkable discoveries and recoveries from the frontiers of neuroplasticity*, Penguin Books.

transformation: your brain on pain[2]. Essentially, these authors' ideas confirmed my own idea that because my spinal nerve was stuck in a feedback loop, it would not necessarily change of its own accord. That nerve would continue to send pain messages, so my best option was to address the pain at the receiving end: the brain. All of these authors and researchers used neuroplasticity to address pain.

Neuroplasticity is the brain's ability to change itself. The science of neuroplasticity is in its infancy. Up until recently, scientists thought that an adult brain couldn't change. However, there is a small amount of research being done about brain changes in chronic pain. I combined these emerging ideas about the brain's ability to change with my own occupational therapy training. I looked at pain as a function of habits and patterns, and I developed strategies to use thoughts and emotions, the physical and social environment, and activities to force the brain to move its attention away from pain.

Right from the beginning of using these strategies, the activities and behaviour changes made sense,

....
2   Moskowitz, M. H. and M. D. Golden (2013). *Neuroplastic Transformation: Your brain on pain*, Neuroplastix.

and over time, my pain reduced. However, it was not all smooth sailing. As you will see later in this book, I talk about activities that interrupt the brain's focus on pain. Unfortunately, many of these activities are seen as a bit old-fashioned. I do not mind telling you that my friends laughed when I would recount my exciting Saturday night of embroidery, or how my extreme creativity and experimentation resulted in a freshly baked, yet inedible, cake going straight into the rubbish bin. To be honest with you, at times I felt a bit silly and childish, such as when I would spend a whole afternoon colouring in with pencils. But I figured that the pain was taking up my time and energy already, so I had nothing to lose in trying new things to get rid of it. Interestingly, my feelings of being silly or of wasting my life subsided over time and were replaced with an increased sense of control. I felt like I was taking control over my life, and hopefully over the pain, and I hadn't felt like that since before that day in my office, marking those pesky assignments.

Taking myself out of my physical and social comforts was the final step for me in defeating my pain. It was a difficult time when I started to challenge my habits around pain. The pain cave, as I have come to call it, is comfortable: that is the whole point. (I will talk about this a bit later in the book.) Coming out of the pain cave was essential for me. Changing the habits and patterns of how I held onto pain released me from its grip. I refocused my brain away from pain, and I changed habits of place, thought, emotions, and actions.

Sitting here now, as I write this chapter, my chronic pain has gone.

It left about a year ago, but it took me a while to notice because it disappeared so slowly. The pain would go for a day, and then for a few days, a few weeks, and before I knew it, I had to concentrate hard to remember the last time it had troubled me. But I need to be careful because I still have the odd bout of acute belly pain, which is usually due to me not paying attention to the subtle body messages designed to make me move. However, overall, my current level of pain is a huge win.

I decided to write this book to share these concepts. Throughout the book, I talk about my pain and the strategies I used to change how pain messages were processed in my brain. I created a plan for myself, and I will give you examples from my plan that might inform yours. I want you to take the ideas that are useful to you, rewire pain processes in your brain, and reclaim your life.

How to use this book

I wrote this book for anyone in chronic pain. It doesn't matter what is causing your pain, because the techniques outlined in this book address the pain message at the level of the brain. They focus on the 'end-user' of that pain message, not the originator.

To help you understand how you can change the 'end-user' of pain messages, I have used neuroscience research and evidence in writing this book, but I have tried to put research reports and neuroscience jargon into everyday language. The aim of this book is to bring this research to non-medical, non-science people, so I have kept the technical details about the mechanisms that the brain uses to change itself to a bare minimum – just to the facts you need to know to enable you to make relevant changes in your life. And I have done that for one reason: living with chronic pain is hard. You already have enough to cope with without trying to wade through dry research and theory to find some relief from pain.

I know that because I have lived it.

I have divided this book into three parts. Parts 1 and 2 give you all the theory and explanation, and Part 3 provides tasks aimed to help you create your own plan to rewire your brain's response to pain. Here is a bit more about each section:

Part 1

In the first part of this book, I look at why people experience acute pain. I also describe how acute pain can easily slide into the lifestyle of chronic pain. Then I delve into the science explaining how chronic pain causes physical changes in the brain. Specific brain areas fire up when they receive messages about acute pain. These same areas continue to fire up with chronic pain messages. They become so focussed on processing chronic pain that they lose their focus on other tasks for which they are responsible. I identify eight areas of the brain that process pain and look at the other functions they are supposed to be doing. Finally, in this section, I begin to look at how the brain pathways associated with pain can be changed, and my pain management strategies begin to take shape.

Part 2

In Part 2, I describe the concepts and research about habits and brain pathways of chronic pain. We look at the habits of behaviour, thought, and emotional responses that you may have started in an effort to manage your acute pain. I explain how sometimes, when that acute pain slips silently into chronic pain, these same habits may be the things that keep you firmly rooted in the pain lifestyle. Without realising it, you could be limiting yourself and unintentionally encouraging your brain to be on alert for pain.

Part 3

Part 3 provides you with a guide to putting together your own pain management program. The two goals of the program are to weaken brain pathways that process pain and change pain habits. To do that, the program focuses on behaviours and actions, with the aim of refocussing the brain and changing the habits and brain pathways of chronic pain.

- **Steps 1 and 2** will guide you through targeting the areas of the brain that are focusing too much on pain. In these steps, you begin to take action to disrupt and redirect the attention of brain processing areas.

- **Steps 3 and 4** will guide you through spotting your own pain habits and developing different, more positive habits. Changing habits was the final step I needed to break free of the pain lifestyle.

- **Step 5** gives you some ideas of how to adapt your strategies to suit fluctuating pain levels.

- **Step 6** gives you a framework to put all of these strategies together, into a plan that you can refer to and share with your friends to get much-needed support.

Hints and tips

There are a few things to know when using the techniques outlined in this book.

Firstly, it is important to remember that there are no quick fixes for chronic pain. You and your brain have taken at least a few months, sometimes years, to unintentionally create and cultivate this chronic pain lifestyle and associated brain pathways. Change takes time, and the amount of time depends on how focussed you are in addressing your habits and patterns. It took me six months to climb out of pain, and considering I was developing the strategies as I went along, I think this was a reasonable amount of time. When you use the techniques and strategies outlined in this book, you need to play the 'long game'. As you will realise after you read the sections on brain changes and neuroplasticity, the purpose of the activities and strategies in this book are to create long term change.

I have made suggestions for suitable activities and strategies, but this is not an exhaustive (or even a prescriptive) list. If you start an activity or strategy that causes or increases your pain, stop immediately and adapt it or replace it with a different one.

Secondly, there is no need to change your medications when using these strategies. Please, NEVER, NEVER, NEVER reduce or stop taking any medication without talking to your doctor first.

You may find that you rely on your pain medication less over time, which is probably going to be a gradual process. In fact, as I sit here now, with one year's distance between me and my chronic pain, I am not sure exactly where my pain killers are. I just slowly stopped needing them.

Now, if you are anything like me, you might be trying a whole lot of strategies, plans and treatments at the same time. I was so desperate for pain relief that I grabbed at anything that came my way. So, if you are using treatments like acupuncture, diets, or anything else, please feel free to continue.

And finally, if you haven't already, please visit your doctor to have a thorough assessment of your pain. If there is an easily treatable cause, I would grab that treatment with both hands if I were you. However, if your pain is caused by nerves, like mine was, then you might find a cause, but no useful treatment. Please don't let that stop you from taking control of your brain.

I created these strategies and present them to you in the hope that you can take charge of your life and control your pain.

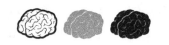

Part 1

PAIN PATHWAYS

Part 1 describes the science and research about the brain's role in pain. This is the foundation on which my pain management strategies are based. In this part, I explain how acute pain can become chronic, altering the wiring in your brain in the process. Then, we take a look at brain plasticity as it relates to pain. Finally, I explain the four activity strategies I used to defeat pain.

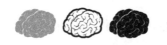

Chapter 1

Sliding into chronic pain

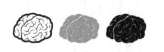

THE STRATEGIES AND IDEAS outlined in this book can be used regardless of the cause of your chronic pain. My pain resulted from damaged nerves, but you might have pain as a result of damaged tissues from a longstanding injury, or even pain that has the dreaded description of 'no known cause'. Because this book addresses pain messages at the brain level, focussing on the 'end-user' of pain messages, the original cause of pain is less relevant.

In saying that, learning about the causes and the processes of pain can provide relief from anxiety and fear associated with pain. but please note, I have not gone into great detail in my description of these complex worlds of pain. I want to give you strategies and plans to help you manage your pain, so I have restricted the explanation to what I think is essential to make sense of my ideas

There are some great books which explain pain mechanisms, such as Butler and Mosely's *Explain pain*[3]. I urge you to get a hold of Butler and Mosely's book to understand more fully what is going on in your body and brain when you are in pain. In the meantime, here is a brief description of what happens and how easy it is to slide from an incident of acute pain to a chronic pain lifestyle.

I think that chronic pain forced me to change my life without me even noticing it was happening.

Acute pain

Pain is a natural phenomenon. We need it for survival. Pain's main goal is to alert us that something potentially dangerous is happening, and that we need to protect ourselves. Pain sends a strong message to our brain that something is wrong, in effect, it immobilises us by forcing us to stop what we are doing. Stopping our actions allows pain to protect us from further damage.

....

3 Butler, D. S. and G. L. Moseley (2013). *Explain Pain* 2nd Edn, Noigroup Publications.

When you hurt yourself, such as stubbing your toe on the coffee table, an electrical signal travels along your nerve fibres to your brain to alert you that something painful has happened. This is called Nociception, and this is only the first part of the pain story.

Sending a message is only useful if it is received. The most important part of the pain story is the bit that happens next – your brain receives the message. Basically, there can't be pain without the brain interpreting and processing those pain signals. That is, if the brain ignores those signals, you will not feel pain.

Have you ever wondered how an Olympic gymnast carrying an ankle injury can run full pelt, majestically backflip across the entire mat and land with a smile? Well, most likely, that athlete's brain is simply too engaged in her routine and too focussed on winning the gold medal to listen to any non-tumbling related signals.

For regular, non-Olympic folk, this same principle applies, but it is harder to override the pain signals. Interestingly, however, these pain signals are overridden when you have an anaesthetic. During an anaesthetic, the perceptive part of your brain is turned off, so the pain signals go unnoticed. That's why surgery only hurts after it is finished (provided you don't wake up in the middle of the procedure, that is).

Without anaesthesia (or the chance of winning a gold medal), your brain is more likely to act on pain signals. It will send messages to your body to do something to protect yourself. The specific action that you do to protect yourself will depend on where you feel the pain, but overall, your brain is trying to achieve the main goal of acute pain, which is to force you to stop doing whatever it is that is causing damage.

Let's say you are walking on the beach and misjudge your footing in the soft sand. In a burst of clumsiness never seen on 'Baywatch', you fall over, twisting your ankle. Suddenly, you feel a sharp pain shooting up your leg. That sharp pain is the signal for your body to stop and protect yourself.

The sharp pain stops you from standing up. Then, the tissues around your ankle begin to swell, protecting the joint more by restricting any movement. The swelling also increases the blood supply to the ankle, bringing white blood cells to mop up the damaged tissues. Muscles surrounding the area contract, further protecting the ankle from movement.

Your body mounts a stress response because it is mobilising its defences, just in case you need to flee or fight to survive. Your blood pressure rises, which might cause you to feel faint. Your digestion stops, or at least slows down, because your body does not want to waste energy digesting your lunch when it might need those resources to go into your muscles to run or fight. And, your immune system focuses on the injury, which means there is less energy left to fight other infections. Right now, your brain considers your injury more dangerous than any other cold or flu that is floating around. All of these consequences of this initial ankle injury are designed to force you to protect yourself and survive.

At the same time as your body is responding, your mind is trying to make sense of what is happening and is assessing the environment for danger. You might feel fear (did I mention it is the depths of winter, and the beach is deserted?). Anger might bubble up, directed at yourself, the beach clearers, or even the sand. Both of these reactions are designed to heighten your awareness and prepare you to run or fight to survive, if required.

All of this is perfectly fine and natural ... in the short term. We develop a strong pain response because we need to pay great attention to acute pain. Pain is unpleasant, but it also has the noble purpose of protecting us. Acute pain gets the immediate attention of our brain, and paying attention and acting accordingly is rewarded by survival. Generally, we are also rewarded when the pain stops a few hours, days or weeks after we cease the activity or action that caused it in the first place.

The problem lies when this attention remains – when acute pain slides into chronic pain.

Chronic pain

Given that the purpose of acute pain is to warn us of danger, it would be logical to think that once the immediate danger has passed, our brain would stop the warning signal, let go of the pain and life would go back to normal. However, for reasons that we still do not understand, some people, including myself, slide into chronic pain.

Chronic pain is generally defined as any pain lasting longer than 12 weeks. It can be caused by many conditions, and contrary to what your brain tells you, chronic pain does not always reflect ongoing damage in your body. Even injuries you might consider insignificant or minor can slide into chronic pain. Many times, tissues have already repaired, but the brain still considers that pain is present, and continues to respond to pain signals[4].

In fact, even if you have been in pain for over six months or so, your body has probably already healed. But your brain is still responding to incorrect pain messages sent from the spinal cord or created in the brain itself. This is called neuropathic pain – sometimes called 'central pain' because the pain is due to the actions of the central nervous system (the brain and spinal cord)[5].

Neuropathic pain is exactly what happened to me. My pain was due to a spinal nerve sending the wrong message and my brain responding to it as if the pain

4 Butler, D. S. and G. L. Moseley (2013). *Explain Pain* 2nd Edn, Noigroup Publications.

5 Doidge, N. (2016). *The Brain's Way of Healing: remarkable discoveries and recoveries from the frontiers of neuroplasticity,* Penguin Books.

had a physical cause in my abdomen. The pain felt as though I was being stabbed, but in fact, nothing at all was happening in my stomach.

Regardless of the initial injury or cause of pain, when acute pain morphs into chronic, lives change.

*Pain persists and activities diminish.
Thoughts get darker as life shrinks.*

This slide into chronic pain usually occurs silently and sneakily. I only noticed I had slid into chronic pain when I looked back on the first six months after my injury. Not everybody has the same path into chronic pain, nor the same lifestyle restriction, but the following is an indication of how easily this slide can happen.

Let's return to the ankle injury on the beach. Here is a scenario that might sound familiar, and it might share some elements with your life:

So, you have twisted your ankle on the beach. Naturally, after you catch your breath lying on the sand, you might hop on your unaffected leg to the nearest rock and sit down. You take the next day or so off work, and then when you do return to your job, you have to use crutches to get around. Obviously using crutches is difficult at work, so you try and alter your work tasks to reduce standing and do more seated activities at your desk.

Using crutches and getting yourself around the workplace is tough, so you cancel the trip to the movies you had planned with your friends. Cooking is also a little tricky when you are on crutches, so you get take-out 'just for a few nights', rest on the couch and catch up on Netflix.

You know that if you walk on that leg, your ankle hurts, but you are not too worried about this minor injury. After all, it is just a sprained ankle.

Fast forward six months and that ankle is still giving you trouble. For reasons that the doctors can't explain, your ankle still hurts, even though no damage shows in any of the tests/X-rays/MRI scans that you have. Maybe if you have more medical tests, the doctors will be able to work it out.

You know there is something seriously wrong with your ankle. It hurts too much for there to be nothing wrong. Sometimes it feels freezing cold and at other times burning hot. At night, you don't get much sleep because it feels like little shots of electricity are shooting up your leg. You increase your pain medication while you wait for the doctors to develop a better plan for you. This increased medication makes you drowsy, but that is better than living with pain.

You cut back on work because you find it difficult to stand on your feet all day, and you have run out of desk-based jobs to do anyway. You are too drowsy from the medication to concentrate for too long, so you stay home most days now, watching TV. You are worried that if this pain does not go away soon, you will run out of money. You even had to cancel your Netflix to save money.

Not only is the 'warning signal' of pain carrying on too long, but so are other bodily responses. The ongoing bodily stress of pain increases cortisol, slowing down your digestion and dampening your immune response to any other infections that come your way. Emotional regions of your brain are affected by the increased cortisol, and life begins to look bleak.

Dealing with chronic pain puts stress on all of your body and increases your risk of other ongoing health conditions. Indeed, further deconditioning and general poor health can result easily from 'the pain lifestyle'. For example, pain and associated swelling of that ankle injury reduces the amount of time you spend standing and your lifestyle becomes more sedentary. This kind of lifestyle puts you at risk of obesity, heart disease and diabetes.

See how easy it was to go from a protective lifestyle to one that is restricted? Now, you may be saying that you still need to protect yourself from damage when you are in chronic pain and not just acute pain, and you are right. However, in chronic pain, we sometimes use those protective behaviours by habit, rather than when they are strictly needed. For example, sure, going to the gym to run on the treadmill wouldn't be smart after an ankle injury, so many people cut out exercise. However, how many people consider that they could exercise by walking gently in the pool? More likely, exercise is cut out altogether in order to be protective.

After a time of chronic pain signals, our brain also becomes extremely vigilant in noticing pain messages.

This combination of protective behaviours and a brain on alert for pain means that many people slip into chronic pain and inadvertently restrict their life, which is exactly what happened to me.

This book might challenge you to think about how you are experiencing pain and whether you have slipped into a pain lifestyle. In Part 2 we will consider how pain may be a result of habit, and how easy it is to inadvertently create a pain lifestyle, but first, let's look at how pain can change your brain (before we make plans for how you can change it back).

Chapter 2

Pain is a brain changer

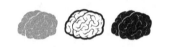

YOUR BRAIN IS THE MOST important organ in your body. It is your control centre, constantly monitoring what is happening and adjusting bodily functions accordingly. And it does this 30 times per second, for every second of your life[6]. It never stops.

So how does pain register in the brain?

Pain messages typically arise in the body, and are carried along nerves, right up through the spinal cord and into the brain. The messages get into the brain via the thalamus. The thalamus is a communication hub. It is central to sending information between the brain and the spine, which in effect means this is where messages are sent between the brain and the rest of the body.

....
6 Moskowitz, M. H. and M. D. Golden (2013). *Neuroplastic Transformation: Your brain on pain*, Neuroplastix.

Pain affects the brain in two ways: by influencing neurotransmitters and by changing the structure of the brain.

Neurotransmitters are the chemical messengers of the brain. When you are in pain, the amount of a neurotransmitter called GABA decreases in both the brain and spine. The decrease in GABA amplifies pain signals, which means you are more likely to feel pain. Less GABA also affects your ability to control your emotions[7].

Another neurotransmitter, dopamine, also decreases when you are in pain. The role of this neurotransmitter is to inhibits pain receptors, meaning that your brain pays less attention to the pain messages. But, if it is decreased in pain, you pay more attention to pain messages. It's a vicious cycle.

Dopamine is not just a neurotransmitter for pain. It is released also in moments of pleasure. When there is less dopamine due to pain, there could also be less pleasure and enjoyment of life. Dopamine is also released when there is a promise of a reward

7 Bushnell, M. C., et al. (2013). "Cognitive and emotional control of pain and its disruption in chronic pain." *Nature Reviews Neuroscience* 14(7): 502-511

to come, which could be a protective factor against pain. Increased dopamine level might explain why athletes can continue to compete even if they injure themselves on the field. That elusive gold medal is a significant reward.

Pain changes the structure of the brain too. When you are in chronic pain, your brain is constantly bombarded with pain messages. This onslaught of pain signals causes the brain to adapt by learning new ways to cope with the increased load of processing pain. More and more brain space is 'on duty', dedicated to managing pain, and different neural pathways are created in response to pain messages flooding the brain.

All of this happens without you knowing it. And, until recently, much of this happened without science knowing it too. Changes to brain structures and pathways happen through a newly identified phenomenon, known as neuroplasticity.

Neuroplasticity

We used to think that an adult brain was set and it couldn't change. However, recent advances in neuroscience showed that concerted and consistent actions can lead to changes in the brain. The ability for the brain to change in response to messages from our senses (including pain messages), our purposeful actions, our beliefs and emotions, stress and traumatic events is called neuroplasticity.

Neuroplasticity is a part of our lives. Every time we learn a new skill, typically by repeating the actions over and over, we are changing our brains by creating new pathways for electrical signals.

The basic idea of neuroplasticity is that repetition creates strong electrical pathways in the brain, while avoiding other activities can decrease the strength of other electrical pathways[8]. Neuroplasticity is the epitome of the old phrase 'use it or lose it'. Learning new skills and repeating actions cause actual anatomical changes in the brain as electrical pathways are created or pruned because of lack of use. In short, brains are wired and rewired by what we do.

....
8 Doidge, N. (2016). *The Brain's Way of Healing: remarkable discoveries and recoveries from the frontiers of neuroplasticity*, Penguin Books.

Neuroplasticity is a response to repeated actions or stimuli. For the most part, a brain that changes to adapt to frequent messages is handy, but it might surprise you to know that plasticity is not always for our benefit. Constant pain messages strengthen neural pathways of pain-processing. That is, as pain becomes more prominent in our lives, the pathways processing the pain in our brains become stronger.

The repetition of pain messages in chronic pain strengthens the brain's pain-processing pathways[9]. So, our brains become vigilant to any threat of pain, and ready to fire up at the mere whiff of an ouch. In some ways, our brain's response to chronic pain messages can be thought of as a new skill, repeated over and over, until it becomes a habit. Your brain has learnt to respond to pain ... but a little too much. Pain has become a habit (more of this in Part 2).

Neuroplasticity due to pain is a double whammy. At the same time as pain pathways are strengthening, pathways of other activities are typically shrinking. We 'lose' the other pathways, or at least, they become

....
9 Arden, J. B. (2010). *Rewire your brain: Think your way to a better life*, John Wiley & Sons.

weaker, and then pain is the biggest thing on our mind ... literally.

When our lives shrink into a pain lifestyle, decreased activities and restricted social and physical environments provide fewer alternative stimuli for the brain. The brain has free reign to concentrate on pain.

Our knowledge of how the brain can change is in its infancy. Exploration into how individual activities change the brain are still a little way off on the research horizon. It is only recently that science has been able to examine the effects of our thoughts, behaviours and actions on brain structures. Improvements in technology now allow researchers to peek into the brains of people when they are in action, thinking, and in chronic pain.

With an increase in medical imaging technology, scientist can now see what areas of the brain fire up during activities, and even when an individual is in pain. This new knowledge opens up new possibilities for changing the brain. The first clue in how we can use the brain to defeat pain can be seen if we explore the idea of 'dual processing.

Dual processing

The brain's ability to use one area for a range of different functions is called dual processing. Our brain is put together in a miraculously clever way. It needs to coordinate many processes at once while being packed into a tiny space inside your skull. That means that it needs to be space-efficient. Certain areas of the brain are responsible for different actions, thoughts, processes, or for managing stimuli that come from our senses. To get the most out of limited space, each area or small section of our brain is responsible for quite a few of these functions.

In pain, it works like this. When you experience acute pain, that pain is processed in specific brain areas. But, in addition to processing and managing these pain signals, those brain areas have other functions, such as regulating our emotions or planning our actions. The short-lived nature of acute pain makes it easy for brain areas to temporarily switch to processing pain messages while maintaining all the other things they need to do. In acute pain, this system of dual processing works well.

However, if the burden of processing pain is consistently felt in these areas, such as when you have chronic pain, we strike a problem. When the various brain areas are busy processing pain, they have less ability to do their other designated activities. The energy and neurones available for non-pain activities are simply unavailable, so the pain pathways in those area of the brain take over.

It might be easier to explain the concept of dual processing if we think of the brain as a collection of little factories.

Our brain is a bunch of factories

Imagine that your brain was an industrial city. A hive of activity. Areas of the brain are separate little factories, and each little factory is responsible for manufacturing certain goods or coordinating specific services. For example, as you are reading this book, factories are busy at work keeping your head still and firing up the muscles in your arm and hand to hold the book. A factory is turning light from your retina into electrical impulses as you read the words on this page. Another factory is making sense of those impulses and interpreting the words. Yet another factory is fitting the ideas and concepts of those words with your experiences. Any emotions you experience as a result of what you are reading are being generated and processed in other factories. As you can see, many factories need to coordinate and do their share even for the most routine of activities.

There are some certain factories that have a sideline in processing pain. If we are lucky, they are only called into action to do this every now and again, in acute pain. In acute pain, extra factory workers (known as neurones) are recruited temporarily from their usual activities to undertake the sideline tasks of processing and managing pain. Because these workers are taken from the main factory tasks, the other outputs and purposes of that factory temporarily slow down or stop. Fortunately, in the short term, there is minimal disruption to the usual factory purpose. After acute pain dies down, it goes back to business as usual at the factory.

But what happens when the pain continues, stealthily moving from acute to chronic pain? What happens when those factories are called on to process pain more and more?

Well, simply put, the sideline job takes over from the main goods production. More and more of the factory workers (neurones) are recruited to manage the influx of pain messages. More and more of the factory floor (brain space) is dedicated to managing pain, and less space is allocated for producing the main goods of each of the factories.

Factory processes (neural pathways) are altered to focus on pain, taking the emphasis away from business as usual. In short, the sideline becomes the main job.

Frequent or constant pain messages wire up the brain to dedicate more and more space to processing pain. That means that constant pain messages cause the brain to dedicate more 'factory floor' and 'factory workers' to processing pain. In fact, in acute pain, only 5% of space in relevant brain areas is dedicated to pain-processing. In chronic pain, however, that goes up to 15 to 25% of the space in those individual factories[10].

But, what do I mean by the "relevant" brain areas? Well, not all of the brain processes pain. Next, we will look at which areas of the brain are involved in

....
10 Moskowitz, M. H. and M. D. Golden (2013). *Neuroplastic Transformation: Your brain on pain*, Neuroplastix.

processing pain, which gives us our second clue as to how to fight it.

Which brain factories process pain?

Neuroscientists have discovered that there are 16 areas of the brain that are involved in processing pain messages[11]. Eight of these areas are in the conscious part of the brain – the part that we can influence by our actions, thoughts, or behaviours. These are the ones we are going to focus on because we can take control to rewire them.

I am going to talk about these conscious eight areas, but don't worry – this is not a science course. I have included a picture of the brain, just FYI. I will simply tell you a little about each area shown on the illustration, and talk about what other particular talents and responsibilities they have. Remember, in addition to these other functions, all these eight areas also are involved in processing pain messages.

....
11 Moskowitz, M. H. and M. D. Golden (2013). *Neuroplastic Transformation: Your brain on pain*, Neuroplastix.

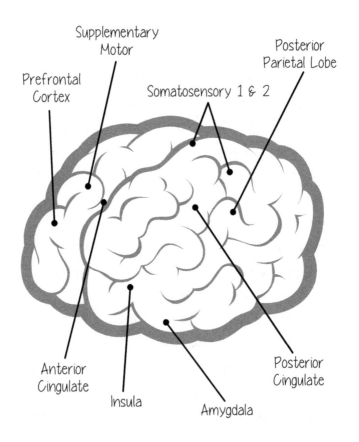

Prefrontal cortex

The prefrontal cortex is where many of the higher level cognitive (thinking) functions of our brain take place, such as memory, problem solving, planning and decision making. It is the part that enables us to be creative, take action, and balance our emotions. It is the area in our brain that is stimulated when we have an intuitive spark. Reasoning and rational thought also lives here.

An interesting role of the prefrontal cortex (along with another area, the insula, which is mentioned a little later) is to decipher mirror neurones. Mirror neurones read the experiences of others and relate them to our own emotional and physical experience – you could almost consider them the building blocks of empathy and the foundation of connecting with others. For example, seeing someone else perform a movement that you would find painful can actually cause you to feel pain[12]. Think of when you have watched a 'funny' video of a ball landing in someone's groin. I bet you groaned, winced, and probably crossed your legs. Well, that wincing, etc, was inspired by your mirror neurones.

....
12 Butler, D. S. and G. L. Moseley (2013). *Explain Pain* 2nd Edn, Noigroup Publications.

Somatosensory areas

These areas play an important role in acute pain by quickly noticing when we are doing damage to our bodies and adjusting our actions without using the other higher thinking areas of the brain. For example, if you put your foot into a scalding bath, touch, temperature and pain sensations fly through these areas of the brain, and you quickly respond by pulling your foot out, all without thinking about it.

These areas also decipher the input received from our senses. As well as temperature and touch, these areas receive information about pressure and vibration. Also, they are involved in understanding of your body position, and the sensation of movement.

Anterior cingulate

The anterior cingulate comes into play when we are trying to concentrate, focus and problem solve. It helps us to control our emotions and detects conflicts with other people.

Posterior parietal lobe

This brain area has some responsibility for interpreting information from our senses and putting meaning to this input. The posterior parietal lobe is particularly interested in interpreting visual and auditory perception. It also contains mirror neurones.

This lobe also has a responsibility for enabling us to locate our body in relation to external space. That is a skill which is used in such everyday activities as placing yourself on a chair or walking on a thin pathway.

Supplementary motor areas

The supplementary motor areas are responsible for organising and planning your movements. Just like a control tower plans and organises planes coming into land, your supplementary motor areas coordinate your actions to create functional movements.

Amygdala

The amygdala is the centre of our 'fight or flight' response when we experience a sudden threat, such as a sabre tooth tiger sneaking up on us from the bushes. In these circumstances, this part of the brain takes over decision making and quickly get us to safety without us having to think about it. However, as you can imagine, problems arise if this area is still active when the immediate threat has passed.

Prolonged amygdala activity is what happens in chronic pain.

As well as coordinating the fight or flight response, this brain area is responsible for our emotions, emotional memory, emotional response, pleasure, sight, smell, and regulating emotional extremes.

Insula

We have an insula buried deep in each brain hemisphere, and up until recently, they were thought to have little function. The insula, like the prefrontal cortex, contains mirror neurones, helping us to connect with others and have empathy. It is also involved in self-soothing, which is being able to regulate emotional responses, and to quieten the fight or flight messages coming from the amygdala.

The insula appears to attach emotional and physical meaning to what is happening in the body. It is also involved in sensing temperature and itch sensations, emotional self-awareness, sensual touch, and disgust.

Posterior cingulate

The posterior cingulate is responsible for visuospatial cognition, which provides the building blocks of spatial awareness. This area is also responsible for autobiographical memory retrieval, which you can think of as reminiscing.

After reading this chapter, I am sure that you can see the potential of neuroplasticity. I hope you are as excited to tackle your chronic pain as I was when I first heard of it.

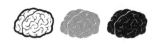

Chapter 3

Rewiring the brain
to untangle pain

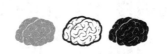

NOW THAT WE KNOW HOW the brain changes in response to chronic pain, we are half way there to changing it back. If the brain can create strong pathways to respond to pain, by using the same techniques of repetition and learning, we can rewire it to de-emphasise these pain messages.

Our goal is to prune the overzealous pain-processing pathways and to get those little pain-processing brain back to focussing on their main role again. By forcing those brain areas to focus on what they are supposed to do, less workers (neurones) and less of the factory floor (brain space) is dedicated to managing pain. And the way to stop using those pathways is to disrupt them by crowding them out with new ones in those same brain areas.

Creating conditions for rewiring

Our strategy for using neuroplasticity and rewiring the brain is to weaken pain-processing pathways and to strengthen different pathways in the same brain areas. We want to build connections between neurones to disrupt pain processing by shifting our brain's attention.

However, not all new actions or tasks we undertake result in neuroplastic changes in the brain. As you can imagine, we are doing new actions every day. If all those actions caused neuroplastic change, the brain would never settle, pathways would not have a chance to strengthen, and actions would not become automatic habits.

The adult brain is selective about when to allow changes and lay down new pathways. Changing the brain requires certain neurotransmitters, or brain chemicals, to be released. For most of the time, these transmitters are in short supply and neuroplastic processes are dormant. However, in certain circumstances, these brain chemicals are released and changes in the brain can occur.

To create changes in our brains, we need to create the right conditions. Much like trying to grow a plant, you need to start with the right soil and nutrients, and then add the extras like sunshine and water. Ok, I've gone off on a little tangent there, but you get the idea. The following circumstances encourage neuroplasticity.

When you are working towards a meaningful task or goal

Your brain needs a reason to lay down a new pathway and remember a sequence of actions. It is not interested in changing to accommodate tasks that are not meaningful and might never be repeated. The brain is working on the premise that there is no point creating a pathway if the task doesn't matter to you, because you might not ever do it again.

Importantly, a meaningful task is one that is a goal for you, it does not need to be a goal that others think is important. For example, think of all those people in the Guinness Book of World records for obscure, bizarre activities. The guy who shelled the greatest number of peanuts in a minute would have practiced and trained, and his brain would have changed as the neural pathways devoted to that activity strengthened. We might think competitive peanut shelling is a waste of time, but clearly that guy thought otherwise, and his brain changed accordingly.

When you are concentrating on the task at hand, and you are paying close attention to your actions

We all know that the harder you practice, the better you get. That is because you are concentrating and trying to improve, and your brain is paying close attention, and coordinating the right sequence of neurones.

When you are faced with something new or unexpected

Neuroplastic activity is heightened in new or unexpected situations. This is likely to be a throwback to our primeval, caveman selves, when we constantly needed to learn and remember what we did to escape danger so we would have pathways ready for action if we faced that dangerous situation again.

In short, the brain allows change when it decides that you are doing something important, and it considers change to be in its best interest.

If the activity doesn't matter to you and you don't put in any effort, the neuroplastic mechanism will not kick in, and nothing will change.

So, the best activities for neuroplastic changes are tasks that are satisfying and rewarding, but also are a bit challenging. If they involve an element of something new, that adds an extra incentive for the brain to create new pathways.

Disrupting, not distracting

Distraction techniques have been part of pain management plans for many, many years. Distraction techniques include watching television, going for a walk, or almost anything that attempts to capture your interest and distract your attention away from the pain. The activities I suggest in this book, however, are not there simply to distract you. I have used my occupational therapy training to analyse activities and tasks, determining the neurological skills required for each one, such as creativity, planning, and body movement. The activities I suggest aim to disrupt pain processing brain areas by redirecting them to their other processing functions.

Firing different neurones together will create new brain pathways. We are not just distracting your mind away from the pain; we are using neuroplasticity, in the form of pain competitors, to create new pathways and change the structure of your mind. And that brings us to the third clue that shows us how to rewire our brain. That of competitive processing.

Competitive processing

In the early days of neuroscience, 1949 to be precise, Donald Hebb introduced a principle known as the Hebbian theory[13]. His theory can be summarised in the phrase, 'neurones that fire together wire together'. That is, repeating actions that stimulate certain neurones to fire at the same time mean that they get used to firing together. What does that mean for pain management? Well, two things:

Firstly, this rule explains how repeated pain messages stimulate certain neurones, and over time, pain responses becomes stronger. Maybe this has happened to you. In the early days of your chronic pain, could you do more than you can now? Could you walk further, sit for longer, tolerate temperature

13 Hebb, D. O. (1949). *The Organization of Behaviour*, Wiley

changes better? If the impact of pain on your life seems to be getting worse over time, your brain's pain responses might be getting stronger.

Secondly, the Hebbian theory gives us a way out of pain. Researchers have demonstrated that you can decrease the strength of a brain pathway and disrupt the strength of neurones firing together by engaging in different activities or behaviour that make other groups of neurones fire together[14]. That is, taking the brain's attention to a different task decreases the strength of neurones in another task. This is called *Competitive processing.*

For those of us living with chronic pain, this means we can compete with pain by using certain behaviours and activities. Competing with behaviours and activities is the key to how I managed my pain. Each time pain intruded into my life, I disrupted the brain factories' focus on pain by forcing them back to their other responsibilities and functions. I did this through activities, thoughts, and behaviours that used these same brain areas.

....

14 Moskowitz, M. H. and M. D. Golden (2013). *Neuroplastic Transformation: Your brain on pain*, Neuroplastix.

By using competitive processing, we are trying to minimise how much energy and space the brain area has for pain. Over time, forcing the brain to reduce its emphasis on the incoming pain messages significantly reduces pain sensation.

Being relentless in disrupting pain processing means that, eventually, the brain pays less attention to pain messages.

More of this in Part 3, where I help you identify strategies and activities that challenge the pain-processing areas of your brain and encourage those areas to focus on the other responsibilities they have.

Meet the 'pain competitors'

To use competitive processing to diminish pain, we need to engage in tasks, thoughts or behaviours that require the other talents or responsibilities of the brain areas that are busy processing pain. I call these 'pain competitors' because they will be competing with pain, and over time, pain will be the loser.

Pain competitors are specific skills or processes needed for some tasks, thoughts or behaviours. Using my occupational therapy background, I have sorted the talents or responsibilities of the eight key brain areas into related groups of:

- higher thinking

- emotions

- sensory information

- moving and positioning.

Some of these talents or responsibilities pop up in more than one brain area.

Higher thinking

Higher thinking can be described as a collection of all those thinking skills, also called executive functioning skills, that make us human. Abilities such as problem solving, morality and decision making are part of higher thinking, as are planning and creativity. Being able to concentrate on a task and focus your energy towards a goal also fall within this category.

Memory is also an important part of higher thinking. Interestingly, the amygdala brain area, which is involved in pain processing, also plays a part in autobiographical memory – memories you have of your life.

As you can see from the illustration on the next page, most of our higher thinking skills and processes are the responsibility of the prefrontal cortex, which is also a big player in the pain-processing stakes. If we can create new pathways there and disrupt the existing pain ones, we are well on our way to decreasing pain.

HIGHER THINKING

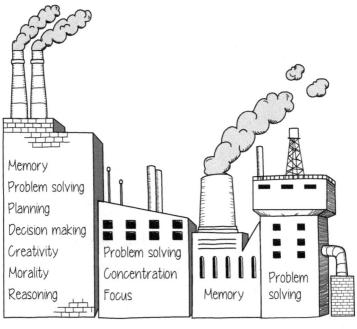

Memory
Problem solving
Planning
Decision making
Creativity
Morality
Reasoning

Problem solving
Concentration
Focus

Memory

Problem solving

PREFRONTAL
CORTEX

ANTERIOR
CINGULATE

AMYGDALA

POSTERIOR
CINGULATE

Emotions

I am sure I don't need to tell you that being in chronic pain means that it is likely you are living with strained emotions, at least some of the time. As we will discuss in the habits chapter, fear and sadness are common companions to chronic pain. It probably isn't a surprise to you then to find out that some of the brain's pain-processing areas are responsible for our emotions too.

The amygdala is one of the key parts of the brain that plays a role in emotions. It also plays a role in pain processing. So, by using competitive processing, we can mobilise our emotions to decrease pain.

What do I mean by 'mobilising our emotions'? Well, look at the illustration of emotional functions of the brain's pain-processing areas on the next page. Actively and consistently challenging existing thoughts and beliefs about the meaning of pain, and our general emotional responses makes new pathways in these areas of the brain. Engaging in pleasurable activities – maybe ones that bring back happy memories – learning to regulate our emotions, and managing stress disrupts neural pathways of pain by strengthening other pathways.

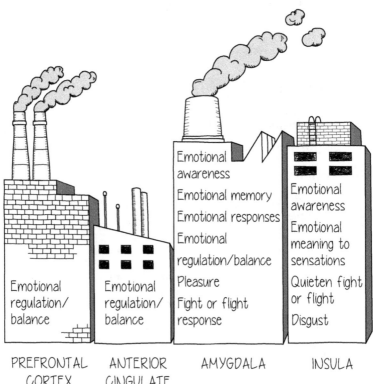

EMOTIONS

PREFRONTAL CORTEX

Emotional regulation/balance

ANTERIOR CINGULATE

Emotional regulation/balance

AMYGDALA

Emotional awareness

Emotional memory

Emotional responses

Emotional regulation/balance

Pleasure

Fight or flight response

INSULA

Emotional awareness

Emotional meaning to sensations

Quieten fight or flight

Disgust

In Part 3 of this book, specifically Step 2, we will identify strategies and activities that use these emotional pathways in the brain. In Steps 3 and 4, we address pain habits, which for some people include habits of thinking and emotional responses

Sensory information

Registering and interpreting information from the senses happens across a smattering of brain areas, including many that are also responsible for pain processing. As you can see from the illustration on the next page, six of the eight identified pain-processing areas that we can influence interpret information from and about the senses. In Step 2, we will identify thoughts, activities and behaviours that rely on information from senses, and that can be used to decrease pain.

SENSORY INFORMATION

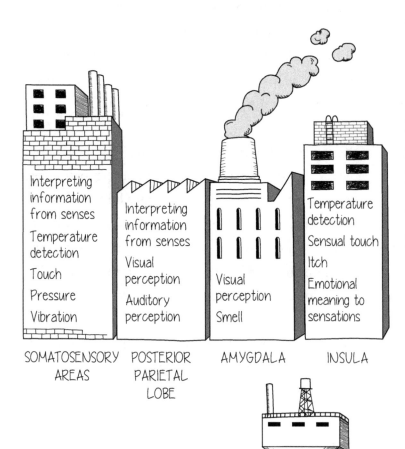

SOMATOSENSORY AREAS

Interpreting information from senses

Temperature detection

Touch

Pressure

Vibration

POSTERIOR PARIETAL LOBE

Interpreting information from senses

Visual perception

Auditory perception

AMYGDALA

Visual perception

Smell

INSULA

Temperature detection

Sensual touch

Itch

Emotional meaning to sensations

POSTERIOR CINGULATE

Visuospatial cognition

Body positioning and moving

When you are living with chronic pain, you are probably living a sedentary life. In our modern world, it is probably a life based around the couch, a computer screen and television. When your body hurts, the last thing you want to do is move. However, moving can be one way to force competitive processing in the pain areas of the brain.

If you look the illustration on the next page, you will see processes that are the building blocks of movement, and they are the responsibilities of pain-processing areas. Navigating your body through space requires your brain to calibrate your body position, interpret the sensation of movement, be aware of external space, and plan and position your world using visuospatial cognition. To sum it up, you need to interpret information from the senses, while planning and organising your movement in order to complete desired physical actions.

BODY POSITIONING AND MOVEMENT

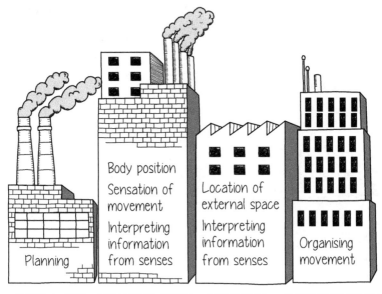

PREFRONTAL CORTEX

Planning

SOMATOSENSORY AREAS

Body position

Sensation of movement

Interpreting information from senses

POSTERIOR PARIETAL LOBE

Location of external space

Interpreting information from senses

SUPPLEMENTARY MOTOR AREAS

Organising movement

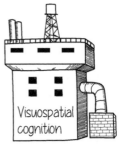

Visuospatial cognition

POSTERIOR CINGULATE

In this chapter, we met the pain competitors and heard about Hebbian's theory of neurones firing and wiring together. All this theory is well and good, but it will remain theory unless there are some simple ways to transfer it into daily life. Luckily, I've done the research and lived the experience, and found the simple ways. In the next chapter, I outline my four main strategies to use pain competitors on a daily basis.

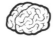

Chapter 4

My four main strategies

I understand if you feel overwhelmed after reading the previous chapter about all the different pain competitors. When I first started using pain competitors, I felt overwhelmed too. Over time, I consolidated all the 'pain competitor' information into four main strategies:

1. moving and being aware of the body

2. being creative

3. bombarding the senses

4. connecting with others.

In this chapter, I explain which areas of the brain are involved in these strategies and their related activities. Additionally, I report on the science and research regarding how some of these activities may influence pain. Then, I give you some ideas on possible actions.

Look, as a researcher and academic, I know the research is a bit light on here, but, I'm writing a book for people who are experiencing chronic pain. I have tried to give you enough research to know that there is evidence out there, but not enough that you have to wade through dry academic writing, especially if you are finding it difficult to focus and concentrate. The goal of this book is not to be a thesis, but to be a mix of information and practical advice.

So, let's get back to the practical advice, shall we?

Up until recently, activities were thought to work by simply distracting someone from their pain. The idea was that whatever it was that you were doing was so interesting that you forgot about your pain for a while. Well, I don't know about you, but when my pain was at its worst, it took up all of my mind and energy. Nothing could distract me. However, over time, engaging in specifically chosen activities did reduce my pain. This happened not by distraction, but by changing my brain's response to pain. By doing specifically chosen activities, those that used the same brain areas as used in pain processing, I could rewire those areas and change how my brain responded to pain.

Remember the competitive processing theory? My idea was to force pain-processing brain areas to concentrate on what I wanted to do, thereby there would be less energy in those areas to focus on pain. My four main strategies all use pain-competitors. When you are creating, moving, bombarding your senses, or connecting with others, the pain-processing areas of your brain are being stimulated.

Let's look at each of my four main strategies in greater detail.

Body movement and awareness

I think it would be a fair bet that you have moved less since your chronic pain developed. Maybe your couch has begun to show a permanent imprint in the shape of you. Or is it your bed where you spend most of your life? I completely understand. During my two years of chronic pain, my bed became my office, entertainment area, even phone conference room (but never Skype, for obvious reasons!)

*But, here is some interesting news —
for some people, physical movement
has been found to reduce pain.*

I can guess what you're thinking. 'That might be ok for *those people*, but I need to stay rigid, still, and unmoving or I might hurt myself.'

Well, no.

Think back to Chapter 1, where I described a path of acute pain sliding into chronic pain. In most situations when pain has hung around too long, there is no new tissue damage, and usually any damage has physically resolved. Your body has healed as much as it can, but the pathways in your brain remain focussed on pain.

In those circumstances, what it comes down to is that pain is simply a mistaken warning signal, not an indicator of tissue damage. So, if tissues are no longer damaged, as long as you start slowly and pay attention to your comfort levels, physical movement is fine. In fact, many activities we think of as physical movement involve some of the same pathways in the brain that process pain. To put it bluntly, moving helps you manage your pain!

Pain competitors in movement

If we're going to delve into the tiny tasks and brain pathways of physical movement, let's not slog it out at the gym. Let's at least take the time to concentrate on something enjoyable. Let me build you a picture:

The light, warm breeze slowly brushes your face as you walk along on the white sand. The sound of the waves lapping on the shore is almost drowned out by the noisy seagulls overhead. Your hat protects your face from the sun, but you can feel its warmth on your bare arms and legs as you steadily make your way along the sea front.

As much as I don't want to disturb that happy fantasy, I am about to pull apart that image into a world of tiny actions and brain pathways. (But, feel free to put the book down and stay by the ocean for as long as you want.)

Did my description of physical activity, which was full of sights and sounds, surprise you? I bet you were expecting me to describe muscles heaving great big weights and limbs flying everywhere in an aerobic frenzy. Well, those CAN be examples of physical activity, but I chose my scenario purposefully. I chose it to make the most of all the available pain competitors. You see, this scenario of walking along the beach would require you to pay attention to two things: information coming into your brain, and the position of your body. If you think back to the chapter on pain competitors, you'll figure out that I am talking about the brain areas that are pain competitors related to sensory information AND body positioning and movement. Two pain competitors in one activity: winning!

Let's break down our seaside scenario.

Below, I describe the role of the main brain areas and pain competitors in that simple walk along the beach. Remember, each of the brain areas I mention is also processing pain. So, using the idea of competitive processing, we can decrease their emphasis on pain if we increase our concentration on other tasks.

During this simple walk, here is what would be going on in your brain. Well, wait a minute. There is a proviso here ...

All activities that you do because you are trying to rewire your pain responses require concentration. Neuroplastic changes won't initiate if you don't pay attention to all your senses and to your body movements. You need to be fully present, not worrying about what you did before your walk or what you need to do after.

Sensory information:

Basking in the sunshine, with the sun on your skin fires up the somatosensory areas with temperature recognition. These areas are also engaged in making sense of the sensation of the soft and silky sand and interpreting the pressure of the sand to make sure you have sure footing. Your posterior parietal lobe is awash with the sights and sounds around you. While your amygdala is also taking in the sights and loving the smell of the salty air.

Body positioning and movement:

This simple walk along the beach really has the supplementary motor areas aglow. Along with sensing temperature and pressure, they are also noting your body position, and the sensation you have of moving your body. Your posterior parietal lobe is joining in the interpretation of information from your senses and locating your body in the physical environment.

Who knew that your brain would be so alert with just a simple walk along the beach? Similar areas of the brain fire with other physical activities and movements too.

When I first started looking into physical movement to disrupt pain-processing pathways, I chose a range of activities, (even though I didn't want to move at all). I wanted something that required slow, precise movements designed to force me to concentrate on positioning my body, while stretching tight muscles. I searched the internet for videos of gentle yoga, wheelchair yoga and sitting yoga, and I found a world of possibilities out there. My favourite was a 30-minute yoga session from an American spinal cord injury association, showing yoga poses in a wheelchair and on the floor. I started with the wheelchair-based poses, and slowly, over the course of a week, progressed to the floor exercises as well.

Initially, nothing really happened with my pain levels, but I began to feel a little like my old self, knowing that I was trying to take charge, and I became motivated to move. Over time, I found that my pain decreased a small amount during a session if I concentrated on each pose. However, if I just 'went through the motions' of the session, I would be able to tick yoga off my to-do list, but I would still have the same level of pain.

After a few months of doing daily yoga (well, almost daily), I knew the poses that had the greatest effect on my pain, and I could do those at other times of the day. At work, on more than one occasion, I locked my office door, got out of my wheelchair, and posed as the 'adapted hanging cobra' on my office floor for a few minutes.

What the research says about pain and moving

In the not-too-distant past, physical activity and movement was considered dangerous when someone was in pain. For example, it was not uncommon for health professionals to prescribe bed rest for back pain. However, a recent Australian clinical guideline[15] recommends exercise for chronic musculoskeletal pain. The guideline authors took a wide approach to movement, and they advised that exercise should be enjoyable, related to a person's goals, and focussed on restoring movement and confidence.

These guidelines are supported by published recommendations by a rehabilitation physician in the journal of the Physical Medicine and Rehabilitations Clinics of North America[16]. The author of that study listed the many benefits of exercise for people with chronic pain, including:

15 Booth, J., Moseley, G. L., Schiltenwolf, M., Cashin, A., Davies, M., & Hübscher, M. (2017). 'Exercise for chronic musculoskeletal pain: a biopsychosocial approach.' *Musculoskeletal care, 15*(4), 413-421.

16 Kroll, H. R. (2015). 'Exercise therapy for chronic pain.' *Physical medicine and rehabilitation clinics of North America* 26(2): 263-281

- improvements in strength and endurance

- improved mood and thinking

- improved bone health

- improved pain control.

She also noted that exercise had positive effects on the brain, including increased sense of well-being and, again, improved pain control.

In earlier research, a group of health academics[17] from Canadian universities reviewed the evidence in studies about resistance training for people with fibromyalgia. Fibromyalgia is an illness that includes pain as one of its symptoms, in addition to fatigue, stiffness, depression and sleeping problems. The authors defined resistance training as exercise that involves lifting weights or using machines or elastic bands that provide resistance to movement.

They ploughed through dry research databases and found 1,800 or so studies, but only five aligned with the goal of examining the research about fibromyalgia

17 Busch AJ, Webber SC, Richards RS, Bidonde J, Schachter CL, Schafer LA, Danyliw A, Sawant A, Dal Bello-Haas V, Rader T, Overend TJ. 'Resistance exercise training for fibro-myalgia.' *Cochrane Database of Systematic Reviews* 2013, Issue 12. Art. No.: CD010884

and resistance training. All of these studies were about women. Overall, the authors reported that the quality of these studies were low, but they did show a decrease in pain for women who participated in resistance training. They concluded that 16 to 21 weeks of resistance training was likely to decrease pain in women with fibromyalgia.

There are plenty more research papers out there, and many others are in the reference list of these three I have mentioned. As movement and exercise are free, I thought they were worth a try, and they worked for me.

Creativity

Don't worry. You don't need to skip this bit if you're not arty. Creativity is not just about representing your burning and tingling nerves in an abstract water colour. Nor do I want you to choreograph an interpretive dance about your gout (although you could if you wanted to).

Creativity, for our purposes, is a broad idea. All I'm talking about when I say creative pursuits are activities that involve you creating something you can be proud of. Creating something from something else helps you see the big picture of how you could transform the world directly in front of you. It could be by being crafty with your hands or clever with the computer. It could be sewing, cooking, painting, writing, knitting, or even upcycling furniture.

I used three creative pursuits to manage my pain. I would do at least one of the three daily, typically just before bed to ease pain and to relax. My main activity was embroidery. No, not your Nanna's style of embroidery, but a funky embroidery (yes, I made up that term just then). I would sew designs based on 1950s pin up models, complete with pointy bras and cheeky grins.

As fun as that was, there were times when my pain levels were too high to concentrate on stitching, or even to sit up. On those days, I would go to my second pain-managing craft choice: adult colouring books. I used these when my pain was bad because I didn't need to concentrate as hard, I could lie on my bed to do them, and I wasn't that invested in the final product. It wasn't a tragedy if my belly suddenly went into spasm, making me flinch and accidentally colour outside the lines.

And then, there were those days ... you know the ones. The pain grips so tightly that you try to stay like a statue, fearing to move just in case you make it worse. You can't concentrate much at all. Even television is too complex to follow. You just want to close your eyes and wait for the pain killers to make the world melt away. Yep, those days that, at the peak of my pain, were almost every day. I had a cunning creative pursuit for those days – online jigsaws.

Online jigsaws were brilliant. I downloaded a jigsaw app onto my mini-iPad, which was light enough to hold when I was lying on my back in bed. I was still being creative by concentrating on shapes and colours, manipulating things with my fingers, and trying to create a finished product. But it was perfect because I could put it down if I needed to sleep and then pick it up where I left off. There were no consequences if I made a mistake. The task had a finishing point and goal to work towards. And, most importantly, I was challenging the pain-processing areas of my brain, while hardly moving.

(Just a little aside: I was so excited about my results from using creativity to control pain that I wanted to call this book 'Cross-stitch your way out of pain'. Sadly, that title got a resounding NO from everyone I know.)

Pain competitors in creativity

My profession of occupational therapy has had a bad rap over the past decades, being called 'basket weavers' and 'craft ladies' (apologies for the 'lady' reference to those 7% of male occupational therapists). The profession has moved away from creativity in recent years. However, it wasn't until I started researching brain function that I saw the neuroplastic potential of craft and creative pursuits, and I began to appreciate the pioneering occupational therapists with their weaving workshops.

Many craft and creative pursuits require a similar set of skills, so they use similar areas of the brain. In general, creative activities require you to generate new ideas, to look beyond the individual components and imagine the possibilities. They involve thinking outside the square and ultimately creating a finished product. Many times, craft and creative activities require small repetitive movements and fine motor control of the fingers (think needlecraft), and because of this, they require concentration.

Let's use knitting as an example, and we will delve deeply into what our brain does when we whip up a pastel pink bed jacket in 'feather and fan' stitch (or alternatively, make a plain scarf, your choice).

Higher thinking:

Whether you're an expert or a beginner, knitting, like other creative pursuits, involves many skills we associate with higher thinking. Your prefrontal cortex, the area of your brain that is just behind your eyes, is almost pulsing with energy when you knit. It fires up as you let your creativity out (you can see how the balls of wool and needles could combine to make something beautiful), plan your next move (was it needle in and wool through, or needle in and wool over?), problem solve as issues arise (why do I have seven more stitches on this row than I had before?) and make decisions (do I really want that pastel pink bed jacket in 'feather and fan' anyway? Is it too late to make the scarf?). Backing up your prefrontal cortex, your anterior cingulate comes alive when you concentrate and focus on that one task.

Sensory information:

Knitting is a constant dance between what you see happening and how you react. And that dance creates the final product. Your somatosensory areas fire up as you interpret information from your senses, such as vision (does my bed jacket match the picture?), touch (gee, that wool is rough), and pressure (I'm holding these needles with a vice-like grip, and the stitches are tighter than before).

It appears that many pain-processing brain areas can be disrupted with craft activities. So, let's look at what the research says about using creative pursuits to manage pain.

What the research says about pain and creativity

Let's face it; craft is a bit passé or old fashioned. Even the research world has trends, and craft is passé there too. I found it difficult to find any studies of the free-flowing, self-driven, 'make it up as you go along' type of craft. So, then I looked at therapies, such as art therapy, play therapy, and other types of creative therapies.

I found a systematic review from researchers from an institute in the USA that is dedicated to translating research into practice[18]. In that review, the authors reported on 146 randomised controlled trials (the gold standard of research), done by other researchers, about treatments for chronic pain involving artistic/creative therapies. The therapies included journaling/storytelling, music therapy, art therapy, dance therapy, colour therapy and play therapy.

This team reported recommendations for journaling and music therapy. The results

18 Crawford, C., Lee, C., & Bingham, J. (2014). 'Sensory art therapies for the self-management of chronic pain symptoms.' *Pain Medicine*, 15(S1), S66-S75.

are a mixed bag, largely due to the quality of the original research designs. I will talk about both of those two therapies individually, so you can make up your own mind as to their benefits. Please note, I am reporting a very brief summary of this review. If you would like to read the whole thing, you will find the reference in the footnote below and in the back of this book.

Journaling – In the systematic review, journaling was described as writing or telling stories to clarify thoughts and feelings, and gain self-knowledge. The review reported on three studies where journaling was used to manage chronic pain, but they described two of these as being of poor quality.

One study was about cancer pain, the other two were about fibromyalgia. None of the studies reported any adverse or negative effects of using journaling, and only one reported positive effects. The authors reported that even though one study had positive results, they were unable to make any recommendations about journaling as a therapy for chronic pain because of the limited and poor-quality research.

Music therapy – Five studies about music therapy and chronic pain were also reported in this same review. They described music therapy as using the physical, emotional, and social aspects of music to create positive change in a person, and to assist them to reach therapeutic goals.

These studies addressed pain from cancer, osteoarthritis, chronic non-malignant pain, lumbar pain, fibromyalgia, inflammatory disease, and neurological disease. Four studies were of high quality, and one was poor quality, according to the review team. None of the studies reported any negative or adverse reactions. The authors of the systematic review concluded that the majority of high-quality studies found that music therapy was effective in managing pain.

Unfortunately, there isn't much more research out there about creativity and chronic pain. However, as science increases our knowledge of neuroplasticity, I'm sure there will be more out there soon.

Bombarding the senses

When I was in too much pain to move or be creative, but I still wanted to fight my pain, I chose activities that required little movement, but they bombarded my senses. We all have five senses (six if you're Bruce Willis); sight, hearing, touch, taste, and smell. To bombard any of these, I put myself in a position where my brain had to concentrate on the information coming in, even while I was lying or sitting still. These activities needed to be simple, and easy to use.

Touch is sometimes heightened when you are in pain. There is something comforting about a warm, cosy blanket, especially when you are in pain. However, for some people in pain, there is nothing worse than being touched, particularly touching their painful areas. These two different responses show how sensitive and responsive we are to touch, even if we are not aware of it.

Using touch as an example, if you are in the second camp and can't stand touch on your painful areas, don't stop reading now. When we use pain competitors associated with touch, that touch could happen on any part of your body. We are interested in making the mind concentrate on the touch sensation, so it doesn't necessarily matter where that sensation takes place on the body; it's the brain pathway of feeling and interpreting the touch that we care about.

Pain competitors in bombarding your senses

There is just one pain competitor here: sensory information. We interact with the world via our senses. We take in information and interpret what we see, hear, taste, touch and smell. Our somatosensory areas do the bulk of that work. The key is the same every time you use the pain-competitors: put effort into concentrating on the sensations coming into your brain. This will allow the activities to compete with the effort the somatosensory area is putting into pain processing.

What the research says about pain and using the senses

Most of the research about using our senses to manage chronic pain focusses on listening to music. Just as I tried to look beyond research about therapies when I was searching for studies about creativity, I tried to steer away from studies of music therapy here. Music therapy is excellent, and has shown to be useful in pain management, but I wanted to know about the effects of using your sense of hearing, not the therapy surrounding it.

Luckily for us, in 2007, Scottish researchers looked into just that, examining the effect of listening to music on chronic pain[19]. Laura Mitchell and her colleagues at Glasgow Caledonian University wanted to know about the use of music by people with chronic pain, whether they considered this part of their pain management plan, and what their perception was of the benefit of listening to music for pain and quality of life. They sent a questionnaire asking about pain levels, quality of life, and music listening to

19 Mitchell, L. A., MacDonald, R. A., Knussen, C., & Serpell, M. G. (2007). 'A survey investigation of the effects of music listening on chronic pain.' *Psychology of music*, 35(1), 37-57

over 800 people who were registered with a Glasgow hospital pain clinic. Just over 300 people replied.

One result they reported will be unsurprising to any of us who have experienced chronic pain. They found a relationship between pain levels and quality of life. Essentially, the higher the pain, the worse the quality of life. In regard to music, the authors found that distraction and relaxation were the perceived benefits of music. They also found a relationship between how personally important music was for participants and how participants used it to ease pain. That is, music was likely to be used for pain management if music was already important to an individual. This result really brought home to me the need to choose an activity that you like and want to do.

This study's findings are interesting in comparison with an earlier paper from 2004 by two Australian researchers, Diana Kenny and Gavin Faunce. Di and Gav (well, they ARE Australian) wanted to explore the impact of music on mood, coping, and perceived pain, so they did this by comparing the effects of singing in a group to those of listening to music while exercising[20]. People who were enrolled in a hospital pain management program were randomly assigned to either a 30-minute singing group, or another group who listened to a recording of singing while they exercised.

The group who listened to music while exercising showed improvement in measures of mood, coping and pain levels at the end of the intervention. These results are similar to those of Mitchell and her colleagues mentioned earlier[21]. However, and here is the interesting bit, the people who engaged in active group singing showed similar results, but had a much greater improvement in the measure of coping. That is, they, like the previous group, improved mood and pain levels, AND they coped better.

Being in either of those groups was a win-win, but I found that last study

20 Kenny, D. T., & Faunce, G. (2004). 'The impact of group singing on mood, coping, and perceived pain in chronic pain patients attending a multidisciplinary pain clinic.' *Journal of music therapy*, 41(3), 241-258.

21 Mitchell, L. A., MacDonald, R. A., Knussen, C., & Serpell, M. G. (2007). 'A survey investigation of the effects of music listening on chronic pain.' *Psychology of music*, 35(1), 37-57

particularly interesting when you consider the pain competitors associated with connecting with others. The question raised in my mind was, 'Was it the act of singing or was it being part of the group atmosphere that brought about changes in coping?' We may never know, but in the meantime, next is some information about connecting with others.

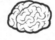

Connecting with others

Pain is an isolating experience. Aside from the physical restrictions that limit your ability to get out and about, you might be isolating yourself inadvertently by limiting your connection with others. You might be so caught up in your pain that it is difficult to see that others need you. You might get angry at friends and family out of the blue, and life may begin to look a bit pointless and stupid. I see connecting with others as a way both to manage pain and to rebuild a life.

It is logical, but not helpful, to shut down your social life when pain becomes the centre of your world.

To me, this sounds like a 'chicken or the egg' dilemma. Given the idea of dual processing, is shutting down your social life a cause or effect of pain? If the brain's focus is on processing pain, you have no brain space left for the processes that are the building blocks of connecting with others. On the other hand, if you're not connecting with others, there is little else occupying those related pain-processing areas, so they may as well concentrate on pain.

Pain competitors of connecting with others

Empathy, or the ability to understand and share the feelings of others, is a role of the prefrontal cortex. We already know that this is a pain-processing area, so having pain is likely to mean less energy and brain space to devote to understanding others. Similarly, mirror neurones are present in four of the pain-processing areas, the prefrontal cortex, posterior parietal lobe, supplementary motor areas, and the insula. As I mentioned earlier, these brain cells interpret the experiences of others and relate them to our own emotional and physical experience. If our brain has less space and energy to relate to our family and friends, we will struggle to connect with them.

What the research says about pain and connections

Just as there is a lack of research into managing chronic pain with creativity, connecting with others is an under-researched area. But we have seen a clue already in Diana Kenny and Gavin Faunce's study[22] comparing pain management of listening to music and singing in a group. (If you missed it, read about it in the research about Bombarding your senses.)

Essentially, these researchers found that research participants who sang in a group showed increased ability to manage their pain than before they joined the group, AND they coped better.

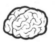

22 Kenny, D. T., & Faunce, G. (2004). 'The impact of group singing on mood, coping, and perceived pain in chronic pain patients attending a multidisciplinary pain clinic.' *Journal of music therapy*, 41(3), 241-258.

Those four strategies, along with addressing my habits, helped me climb out of chronic pain. In Part 3, I walk you through ideas, steps and plans to help you out of chronic pain too. But first we are going to delve into the second part of my approach, which is all about habits.

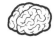

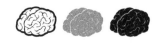

Part 2

PAIN HABITS

Part 2 explores the concepts and research about habits in chronic pain. We look at habits of behaviour, thought, and emotional responses that you may have started in an effort to manage your acute pain, but have since become an everyday part of your life.

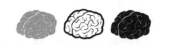

Chapter 5

Pain is a habit changer

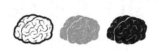

HAVE YOU EVER DRIVEN TO WORK, but couldn't remember how you got there? You didn't think about where to turn left, or which freeway exit to take. It all happened automatically, and you somehow got to where you were going. We have all done it, and it happens because that drive has become a habit.

Habits help us get through our daily lives without wasting energy and time. But sometimes the way we respond to pain has become a habit. Rather than helping, these pain habits keep us trapped in the pain lifestyle.

What are habits?

A habit is a tendency to respond to a familiar environment or situation in an automatic way[23]. With a habit, we respond to something we encounter frequently with automatic behaviours, thoughts or even emotions. Habits are the things we do without even thinking about them. You could say that habits are our unstated rules for daily living because we perform those behaviours, think those thoughts, or feel those emotions consistently and automatically.

Performing a habit over and over creates a pathway of action in the brain. Each time that same environment or situation emerges, the same pathways are used, again and again, until they are well-worn tracks. Relying on well-worn brain pathways frees us up to think about other things. Be honest, when you were driving to work, habitually, without any need to think about where you were going, I bet you were not just sitting there with an idle mind. Were you talking on the phone (hands-free of course!), singing along to a song on the radio, or even practising asking your boss for a

23 Kielhofner, G. (2008). *A model of human occupation: Theory and application*, Lippincott Williams & Wilkins.

raise? Your brain was engaged in other thoughts, while the usual 'get to work' pathways took you through your morning drive.

Habits provide structure in our daily lives. If your usual daily habits are tampered with, it can change your whole day. For example, if you are an early-bird, sleeping in until midday can make you feel groggy all day. If you normally end each day with a nightcap and a warm bath, you might not sleep so well if you go to bed after coming home late from a nightclub. Our habits provide a framework for our day.

Habits are learned behaviours, thoughts or emotional responses. They are typically made up of a group of related activities that are needed to complete a task or behaviour. For example, brushing your teeth is a habit made up of many related actions, which you never really think about, except when you were learning to brush your teeth as a little kid. These individual actions include reaching for your toothbrush, uncapping the toothpaste, applying it to the toothbrush and putting the brush in your mouth – and that is just for starters. With repetition and time, your brain has 'chunked' these tasks together to form the seemingly simple habit of brushing your teeth.

When we refer to "habits", we are usually referring to something called the "habit loop". You can read more about the habit loop in Duhig's book[24]. In my book, I am only concentrating on the habit loop as it pertains to pain.

The habit loop

As complex as habits sound, we create and reinforce habitual actions, thoughts and emotions using quite a simple system of cues and rewards. This system is not that different to a hungry mouse running through a maze, to be rewarded with a piece of cheese. Yes, sometimes humans are that simple.

Essentially, our brain identifies a cue, which starts a familiar sequence of actions, thoughts or emotional responses – a habit routine – which is designed to bring about a pre-determined reward. Every time we respond to a certain cue with that same routine and receive the expected reward, we reinforce a

24 Duhigg, C. (2012). *The power of habit: Why we do what we do in life and business*, London, Random House

habit loop. The more often you complete that loop, the more ingrained that habit becomes.

Let's break down the three elements of habit loops: cues, habit routines and reward.

Cues

Specific stimuli in the environment or a familiar situation that initiates a habit routine is known as the cue. The cue is a hint to the brain to tell it to start a familiar pattern. It is also the signal to the brain to power down and rely on developed automated pathways.

Some cues can be obvious, such as beginning the morning drive. In that example, hopping in your car early in the morning, dressed in work clothes, with your travel mug of coffee might be the cue needed for your brain to switch on the 'get to work' pathways. The rest is automatic.

On the other hand, some cues are hidden from clear view. Only our brain senses the familiarity of a pattern and knows something that we have not figured out yet. Later, I will share with you a cue for a pain habit that slipped below my radar for months.

Habit routines

Habit routines are the most obvious aspects of a habit to spot. These are the behaviours, thoughts or emotions that come about when your brain responds to the cue. When people say that they have a 'bad habit', such as smoking, it is the habit routine of smoking itself that they are referring to, not the cue or the reward.

Habit routines can take many forms. They can be, but are not restricted to, physical actions. You can have a habit in how you structure your daily life, such as a being one of those people who are perpetually busy. You can create thought habits, such as being a Pollyanna and always seeing the positive in any situation. Emotional responses can become a habit, such as if you respond consistently to criticism with anger. You can even create habits in your social and physical environments, such as spending most of your time with the same people, even if they annoy you. Later in this chapter, we will look at these realms of habit routines and see how they relate to chronic pain.

Rewards

Now, you might think that rewards are the obvious element in the habit loop, but rewards are complex.

Like cues, rewards may be perceived by our brain just slightly below the level of our everyday consciousness. What I mean is, if we look hard enough, we can determine the reward that our brain is seeking, but sometimes we need to look harder than at other times.

Let's take an obvious example, such as the habit of eating well. When I eat unprocessed food that I have cooked myself, I always feel healthy and energetic. A simple reward. You would think this simple reward of feeling healthy would encourage me to cook every day. But no. When I have a bad day, eating well is the first thing that goes. On a bad day, my habit routine is to go to a takeaway on the way home from work and pick up something quick, tasty and oh so fatty. The rewards of comfort and treating myself trump feeling healthy. When my brain is triggered by the cue of having a bad day, the rest is a habit routine until I reach my reward of comfort over health.

It might be challenging to even think about it, but I think living a pain lifestyle produces rewards, but some of these are negative. In Part 3, I guide you through examining your own habits around pain, looking at potential negative rewards of the pain lifestyle.

Non-helpful habits

The phrase, 'man is a creature of habit' is not a lie. It illustrates how our lives can be a product of the habit loops we create. We are what we repeatedly do. These simple maxims indicate that our lives can be both improved and restricted by habits. In many ways, habits help us get on with our day, but they can also limit our actions in a negative way.

Habits can keep us stuck. We may be stuck in a habit that we know we need to change. But as we will see, changing a habit means we need to take a long hard look at the cues and rewards, as well as the habit routines.

For example, here is a scenario you may recognise. Have you ever been on a diet to lose weight, but could not resist your usual 3pm chocolate from the vending machine at work? I have and it's almost impossible! (In fact, if I am totally honest, I am sitting here right now with a coffee and a square of chocolate, and it is almost 3pm). You know you should cut down on chocolate, but the cue of the mid-afternoon slump, and the anticipated reward of extra energy from the sugar rush are just too hard to resist. The habit loop overrides your intellect and knowledge of healthy eating.

Sometimes we do not realise we are responding to cues in the environment or situation with a habit routine. Don't believe me? Well, take note of the next time someone gives you a compliment. Do you say, 'thank you' and feel happy, or do you do what most people (at least, most women) seem to do, and say, 'it's nothing really', and downplay the praise? For most of us, we have a habit of responding to compliments with negative self-talk. It sounds illogical, but it appears to be a widespread, self-deprecating habit.

Habits change the brain

Habits are amazing things. They free up our mind so that we can focus on other things and they help us to structure our day. They also maintain our thinking, behaviour and emotions in our standard, usual ways. And the most amazing thing about habits is that they have a physical basis in our brain.

So, what is happening in the brain when we form habits?

As I have mention, there is a phrase in neuroscience, from the Hebbian theory, 'neurones that fire together, wire together'. That means that when we repeatedly do something, the same neurones that are responsible for that action, thought or emotion fire each time. Over time, as your repeated action becomes a habit, these same neurones act together in a coordinated way. In turn, this coordinated action strengthens the neuronal pathways. After a while, all we need to do is simply enter into that habit loop, and those pathways kick in. Then, those actions, thoughts and emotions happen automatically.

Here is a sporting example to illustrate what creating pathways mean. Imagine that you were playing baseball for the first time and learning how to bat. At first, you might find it awkward to hold the bat in the correct position. You might swing, and maybe make contact with the ball, but more likely, you probably hear a swish, feel a blast of air, and see disappointment in your coach's eyes as the pitch goes wooshing through to the keeper.

While you were concentrating on making contact between the bat and the ball, your brain was busy recruiting the right neurones and trying to coordinate them to fire at precisely the right time for the bat to contact the ball. As you practice more and more, your brain gets better at coordinating the recruitment and timing of neurones. Practicing your swing teaches the neurones when and how to fire as the 'hitting the ball' habit routine is formed. As this batting habit routine strengthens, so to do the neural pathways in your brain.

In your second baseball season, most likely, all you need to do is pick up the bat and hold it behind your ear (which acts as the habit cue), and your brain knows what to do next, as the 'hitting the ball' habit routine is initiated. Your brain relies on the well-worn act of knowing the right neurones to fire, and the pathways to activate. I am not saying you would necessarily smash it out of the park, but you would be less likely to disappoint your coach (which could be a habit reward in itself).

However, don't think that these habit routines have to be physical acts only, such as in the baseball example above.

Thoughts and feelings can create well-worn pathways too.

The brain turns repeated actions, thoughts, and emotions into pathways, and in my case, that simple knowledge made me address pain in a different way.

After I had been in pain for about six months, I began to question my daily life. It dawned on me that the chunking of similar tasks into one package of a habit routine, and the use of cues and rewards may be creating pain habits, and thereby stopping my pain from abating. I asked myself, 'What if the activities I use to try to ease my acute pain have become habits that I have carried into chronic pain?' And, more importantly, 'What if these habits were chunked with the processes of detecting and responding to pain in my brain?'

I began to suspect my routines of behaviour, environment, thoughts, and emotional responses were holding on to my chronic pain. What if my pain had become a habit?

Pain as a habit

It is not unusual when someone has an illness or injury that causes acute pain, for them to make subtle changes to their lifestyle and daily activities to manage, and hopefully decrease, the pain. This makes perfect sense and it's the right thing to do. In the beginning, making changes to our daily life allows us to protect ourselves. However, these changes can easily become habits, and it is possible that habits can become a negative influence on our lives.

Habit loops, that is cues, routines and rewards, start as appropriate responses to acute pain. However, over time, as pain become chronic, these habits strengthen the neural pathways that are responding to pain and in turn, shrink our lives.

Simply put, I believe that my chronic pain started as acute pain, but became a habit.

I slipped into many pain habits. Some were harmless, such as my morning ritual of a strong coffee in bed so I could 'ease into the day'. I would typically wake with belly pain and I knew that a hot drink would ease the pain. The reward was easing pain and also staying in bed a bit longer. So, the daily habit loop of making a coffee and taking it back to bed was set. Even now, when I am no longer in pain, this habit is still strikingly difficult to break. In fact, that is how I started the day today. Because this habit has no harmful effects (if I remember to set my alarm for that little bit earlier), I'm not worried about it, and I'm not looking to change it.

Other pain habits I had, however, were harmful to my lifestyle when they were maintained too long. These habits were hard to spot because at the time they were forming, they filled an important need for self-protection. I came to term these 'pain habits'.

The most pervasive of these pain habits, and one that I think most of us share, was the use of social media. When I was in pain, I was sad that other people were out having fun. I felt this most keenly on the weekends. The cue to start this pain habit of trawling social media was that I was lonely and bored at home. I would not spend hours on social media, but I would spend more time there than it was worth. And not just once. I would repeatedly check Facebook or Twitter on my phone to make sure I was not missing out on any new event. The reward that I thought this habit routine was giving me was to see what people were doing, and how they were having fun, and therefore I could still feel part of what was going on. However, in reality, I would look for signs that people were as miserable as I was, and if they were actually having fun, I would feel sadder. So, the cue was understandable, but the routine was off, and then that led to the wrong reward.

The realms of pain habits

That last example of my social media use is a reminder that habits are not only about daily activities or behaviours. They can be about emotions too. My habit around social media was born from the cue of emotions (sadness) and led to the reward of other emotions (actually, still sadness).

Habits can form in many realms, or aspects of our lives. Pain habits have an impact on many areas, but I think concentrating on a few can go a long way in managing pain. The realms that I am interested in are the habits in our daily activities, our physical and social environments, our thinking and our emotional responses.

Pain habits of daily activities, or the pain lifestyle

When acute pain has hung around too long and becomes chronic, our instinct is to continue the immediate protective behaviours we had at the start of the pain. Over time these behaviours become habits and create patterns of brain responses, which continue to feed our perception of pain. This is what I call the 'pain lifestyle', and it is an easy lifestyle to accidentally adopt.

The pain lifestyle is a sedentary one, and increasingly, this is a life focussed around a screen. Screen-based entertainment, such as television or movies, is generally passive so this is a lifestyle where physical activity and exertion are cut back to the bare minimum.

Here are a few scenarios and questions to get you thinking about whether you have adopted elements of the pain lifestyle:

When you first became injured, maybe you stopped cooking dinner because it was too difficult to stand for long enough. So, you started a steady diet of takeaway and frozen dinners. Are you still doing that, even on your good days of less pain?

Maybe you injured yourself playing sport, such as landing awkwardly at netball and tearing the ligaments in your knee. Since then, have you cut out all sports? Even those ones that don't involve putting weight on your knee, such as upper body strengthening or water aerobics?

Maybe you stopped going to work and spent your first few months of pain watching television to pass the time. Even if you have gone back to work since your initial injury, do you still spend a lot of your leisure time in front of a screen?

The 'pain cave' – pain habits of physical and social environments

The environments in which we spend time can become a habit. Maybe that's why they are called habitats. The pain cave is my name for the environmental conditions that I would create to manage my pain when it got too much for everyday life. Think of being cosy in a warm, dark cave. In the acute phase of my pain, the pain cave was absolutely essential to cope with the assault on my body and mind. It was my comfort zone.

Like all habits, the pattern of where we spend time

can have both negative and positive influences on our lives. For example, if we make a habit of going to the gym or walking in the park every night after work, we are more likely to be healthier than if our habit is to slump on the couch. And, to put it bluntly, the 'where' we spend our time influences the 'how' we spend our time. In your pain cave, sitting on the couch, in front of the television, near the snack bowl is a definite health risk compared to being at the gym or the park.

Who we surround ourselves with can become a habit also. I am a big believer in the idea that we become the average of the five people with whom we spend most of our time. That is, we subconsciously pick up the mannerisms, ideas, and behaviours of the people around us. Spending time around enthusiastic, energetic people can make us feel motivated and excited about life even if nothing in our world has changed. We pick up on the habits and patterns of others, so it makes sense to make a habit of spending time with positive people.

The pain cave goes hand in hand with the pain lifestyle. In fact, the pain lifestyle usually takes place in the pain cave. The cave was created by the physical space I was in, the information that my senses were picking up, and the people I was with. The specifics are not that important, but I am sure you will relate to the generalities.

My pain cave

It was quiet in my pain cave, but there was always a bit of noise to try and distract me from pain. Typically, that noise came from a television on low volume. I might have been looking at the screen, but not much of the story was sinking in. In fact, I preferred to watch cooking shows because there was colour and movement, but I didn't need to know the details of what was happening. The cave, mostly my bedroom, was dark with the only light coming from that screen. It was warm in the cave too, usually because I would wear a big cosy jumper, known as 'the sick jumper'. A cup of tea was never far away from the cave, and sometimes, well mostly, if I am honest, a piece of chocolate was my reward to myself to help get through a difficult time.

Even when I was not in pain, but went to bed early because I was tired, entering the pain cave signalled to my brain that we were in pain. The pain cave created the cue for my brain, and pain became the routine. Breaking out of the pain cave was vital for me to manage chronic pain.

After reading my description, take some time to consider whether you have created your own pain cave.

Pain habits of thinking

If you have been in pain for a while and have gone down the medication pathway, you probably know the muddle-headed feeling associated with pain killers. You may have experienced difficulty in putting your thoughts in order and trying to function. Well, what if I were to tell you that the brain-fog wasn't just due to the pain killers? Recent research indicates that pain itself interferes with thinking. Researchers have found that chronic pain is associated with reduced cognitive functions, difficulty with thinking, and it is most pronounced in the areas of memory and attention[25].

So, there we have two good explanations for impaired thinking in chronic pain: medication and the effect of the pain itself. But I have a third possible reason: habit.

Being in pain creates habitual thoughts about your life. For most people, these thoughts typically centre

25 Dick, B.D., Rashiq, S., 2007. 'Disruption of attention and working memory traces in individuals with chronic pain.' *Anesth. Analg.* 104, 1223-1229.

on how restricted they feel their life is. Remember how habits change the structure of your brain? Well, those habitual thoughts about your pain and your restricted life also change the structure of your brain. That's right, your thoughts create and change physical structures in your brain. That's amazing!

The trouble arises if these thoughts create physical structures that feed into a pain lifestyle. For some people, the meaning of pain is catastrophic. Their thinking is one of devastation and of no tomorrow. Let me list a few common thoughts about pain and have a think about whether any have ever crossed your mind:

- My pain is so strong that there must be something seriously wrong with me.

- Even though the tests are clear, this much pain must mean that the doctors just haven't found the cause yet.

- I better not go out just in case my pain comes back.

- I'm going to stop everything until this pain goes away completely. I don't want to risk getting hurt again.

Pain habits of emotions

Emotions, like actions and thoughts, create pathways in the brain. These pathways may also feed into a pain lifestyle. For example, it is not unusual for people in chronic pain to also be afraid, sad, or depressed. No doubt part of that is because of the lifestyle restrictions of pain, but another reason may be that these emotions have become habits of their own.

Emotions of pain have physical causes too. When a pain message reaches the brain, a hormone called cortisol is released. This hormone surges through the brain, placing it on red alert for any other danger. Remember that acute pain is a danger signal in itself, so the brain's logic here is that there might be other dangers nearby that you need to flee from or fight. However, when this hormone is repeatedly awash in the brain, such as in chronic pain, it begins to affect other functions, notably those of the emotional regions of the brain. These regions decrease their ability to self-regulate, and again, memory storage and language abilities are impaired.

You can feel the effect of increased cortisol when you are under stress. You might lose sleep, have difficulty concentrating, become a bit snappy, and feel overwhelmed by life. Add chronic pain to those effects of cortisol, and it is no wonder that we sometimes develop pain habits in our emotional responses.

Fear and sadness are common emotional experiences of people with chronic pain.

Let's look at these two emotions more closely.

Fear

It is not uncommon for the cause of someone's chronic pain to be unknown. A common scenario is that an acute injury just didn't get better in the way it was expected. The pain never really went away, and in fact, it got worse.

Pain without a solid, objective, logical cause can create fear; the fear of the unknown. If your doctor cannot find a reason for your pain, or why it is persisting, it is natural to be fearful. But, if you have been in pain for over six months, the chances are that no further physical damage is happening. The more likely reason for your pain is that your brain is stuck in a feedback loop, as mine was. Research has shown that taking time to study and understand what is happening in the body and mind in acute and chronic pain can reduce fear, and sometimes reduce pain[26].

However, just knowledge alone might not be enough to shift fear. Unfortunately, in chronic pain, the brain can perpetuate this emotion simply by attending to pain. When the brain receives pain signals, the amygdala fires, as we saw in Part 1. The amygdala is also responsible for managing our fears. If the amygdala is busy with pain, it has less energy and space to manage fear and other emotions.

Sadness

Another common emotional response to chronic pain is to feel sad at all the things you have lost, including the life you had planned. After a few months of pain, it would be unusual for you to still be fulfilling all of your work obligations, honouring your family commitments and responsibilities, maintaining your social life, running a household, and generally having a good time. If your experience is anything like mine was, your life will have shrunk around the edges. Some of the shine will have worn off life, and sometimes it is just a struggle to get through a day.

----

26 Butler, D. S. and G. L. Moseley (2013). *Explain Pain* 2nd Edn, Noigroup Publications.

For some people, chronic pain is associated with developing depression, which is an illness unto itself. Many people mistake a bout of sadness for depression. Sadness can certainly be a feature of depression, but that is not always the case. For some people with depression, there might not be sadness or tearfulness, in fact they could be angry and agitated most of the time. A key feature of depression is that people experience what is called anhedonia, which means they get no joy out of the things that used to give them pleasure. Life does not bring any happiness at all.

If you think you might be experiencing depression, please see your doctor or mental health professional. Depression is not a sign of weakness. It is an illness, and it can be treated by both medication and non-pharmaceutical methods. Winston Churchill named his depression 'the black dog'. Learning to tame the black dog will make it easier for you to tackle chronic pain.

If you recognised your life in some of my examples of pain habits, don't be too hard on yourself. It's so easy to slip into a pain lifestyle. After all, at the beginning stages of your pain, you were doing the right thing. Those actions, thoughts and emotions started as self-protection. Now, they have just hung on too long.

In the next chapter, we will explore how you can take back your habits and reclaim your life.

Chapter 6

Taking back your habits

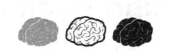

AS WE SAW IN THE LAST chapter, the brain may learn to respond to pain in a 'potentially once helpful, but not anymore' habit loop. In this chapter, we consider how our conscious actions, behaviours and thoughts can be used to teach it another way, and to unlearn this response.

If you want to use the strategies in this book, you will need to move beyond what you thought your limitations were. I don't mean that you need to push yourself into pain; that is never the answer. What I mean is you will need to tackle daily life in a slightly different way. You will need to step out of the pain cave by doing familiar activities in different ways, or by incorporating unfamiliar activities into your life.

To show you what I mean about simple changes to daily tasks to escape the pain cave, let's look at the typical daily task of cooking dinner.

Here's a common scenario, straight from my kitchen: It's dinner time, and I feel a pain all over, but I still have to eat. It has not been one of my good days. Usually, on a day like this one, I would stay firmly in the pain cave. From the safety of the cave, I would reach for the phone and dial up some quick, easy, probably fatty, food delivery service.

However, this time, I pause for a moment and think about how I could break that pain habit. A simple break in that pain habit would be to cook dinner, but how? And why would I bother?

Well, on a basic level, the 'why' could be that I want something that tastes good, but there are also good reasons for me to cook dinner that contribute towards my pain management.

Firstly, cooking is a creative, physical and thinking activity, requiring key brain factories to shift their focus from processing pain to their other responsibilities. With concerted use over time, I could can diminish the strengthen pathways, and crowd out the brain's focus on pain.

Secondly, eating a nice dinner (or, let's face it, sometimes just edible is the target) means that I could achieve a goal that I set for myself. I pressed on beyond what I thought were my limits. Over time, consistently reaching my goals gives my body and mind a signal that I am in control, not my pain.

Finally, a nutritious meal gives my body a better chance of coping with the stress that chronic pain puts on it. I will be protecting myself from lifestyle diseases, such as obesity or diabetes, that can happen when pain restricted physical activity.

But what about the 'how'? Luckily for me, my kitchen is wheelchair friendly. But what about you and your physical needs? Well, an occupational therapist could give you ideas on how to adapt your environment to maximise your physical ability. For example, how about sitting at the dining table to do all of the chopping tasks? Maybe you could perch on a stool while you cook at the stove top? Changing how you do tasks such as cooking allows you to think beyond pain limitations.

As you can see, these ideas are logical, and in many ways, simple.

Rather than taking on a whole new regime of tasks and therapies, I think the best approach is to reframe and adapt your everyday activities into opportunities to break your pain habits.

Consistency in fighting pain habits and weakening the brain's pain pathways is the key.

Addressing pain habits

There is not one simple way to change habits. We develop certain habits to meet specific needs. It stands to reason that some habits will be easier to shift, while others will be more ingrained. Nevertheless, the first step in changing habits is to identify them.

To identify habits, we need to return to the habit loop, to the ideas of cues, habit routines and rewards, discussed earlier. Breaking up a habit into these three components helps to identify what is going on, and why. I will give you a quick overview of what these components might look like in chronic pain, and then some specific examples that you might recognise from your own life.

Spotting the cues

Remember that the cue is the stimuli in the environment or the situation that initiates a habit routine. When you first start to look at your habits of pain, spotting the cue that triggers your habit routine may not be as obvious as you might imagine. Sometimes the cue is an increase in pain intensity, but at other times, it might be something completely different, and seemingly not related to your pain at all. Less obvious cues could come from your physical environment, the time of day, who you are with, and what just happened.

I had a pain habit of which I was not aware for a long time, and it started with a seemingly irrelevant cue. I only became aware of it on one bright sunny day when I was relatively pain-free. I was driving a friend to her home, and when I got out of my car, sat in my wheelchair and reached over to take my keys out of the ignition, I said, 'Gee, my belly is sore'. It was not until she pointed out that I had just told her I was feeling good that day that I realised my belly was not sore at all. That statement was said out of habit.

Over the next few days, I paid a bit more attention to what I was doing, and I noticed that every time I reached and leaned forward in my wheelchair, such as to get the keys from the ignition, the words 'Gee, my belly is sore' tumbled out of my mouth, even if I was not in pain at the time.

The cue was leaning forward. When I was actually in pain, that cue led me to say the truth because the pain in my stomach DID get worse when I leant forward. However, as my pain started dissipating or becoming less constant, leaning forward did not always cause pain.

I was telling myself a lie. The cue of leaning forward then led to the unhelpful habit routine of verbally reminding myself that I should be feeling pain.

As you can see from my example, sometimes the cues are so unlikely that they are difficult to see.

Spotting the habit routines

The habit routine is the most obvious part of the habit loop to spot. It is the behaviour, thought or emotion that you want to change. When people say that they have a 'bad habit', such as smoking, it is the action, or routine, of smoking itself that they are referring to. They are not criticising the cue of break time or the reward of feeling satisfied. It is that specific behaviour of the cigarette in their mouths that they are labelling as bad.

Spotting the routines of pain habits can be both easy and difficult. Habit routines can take many forms, such as routines in thoughts, feelings, habitats and daily activities. The more obvious habit routines, such as going to bed in the middle of the day, are clear to everyone. But other non-tangible routines, such as ordering takeout or being jealous of a friend's success can be harder to identify as a pain habit. Examining your life for routine behaviours, thoughts, or feelings, or even the social and physical environment that you find yourself in frequently can give you clues about your pain habits.

Spotting the rewards

Like cues, rewards can sometimes be difficult to spot. The most common reward that we all seek from pain habits is to stop hurting. You don't need to be a rocket scientist to figure that out. However, there can be other rewards too.

Self-protection is a strong reward at the best of times, but it is accentuated when you are in chronic pain. As we have seen, the purpose of acute pain is to make us stop and protect ourselves. It is logical to see how, in chronic pain, we create habits to continue self-protection. This is not such a bad thing. However, sometimes self-protection can become self-restriction. Taking time to identify and examine the rewards of your pain habits can help you to see if they are healthy rewards or not.

You will need to do some experimentation to identify your rewards because we are often not conscious of the needs that drive our behaviours, thoughts and emotions. In Part 3 we get down to the nitty gritty of this. I will show you how to examine your own pain lifestyle and identify where you can make changes.

Well done. You have got through all of the theoretical explanations. We have talked about the new and exciting world of neuroplasticity. And hopefully you can see the possibilities to help your brain to respond to pain differently.

We have also looked at habits, particularly around the pain lifestyle. It is easy to understand how seemingly helpful actions, thoughts and emotions in acute pain can become tiresome, perpetuating habits in chronic pain.

And now, in Part 3, we will move on to create your plan to rewire your brain and reclaim your life.

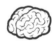

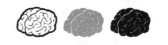

Part 3

YOUR REWIRING PLAN

As promised, here is the step by step guide to rewiring your brain. In this part of the book, we put together your own pain management plan in six steps. The six-step plan will focus on behaviours and actions, with the aim of refocussing your brain to change the habits and brain pathways of chronic pain. I'll start with a summary so you know where we're going with this, then we'll get into it

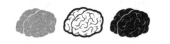

Summary of steps

Step 1

We briefly revisit the brain areas that process pain, (primarily for those of you who skimmed over Part 1). We then consider the other tasks that those brain areas are supposed to be doing, and we identify some pain competitors that disrupt your brain's focus on pain. Remember that over time, activities that use pain competitors can weaken pain pathways, so I guide you to identify specific activities that use pain competitors to challenge the pain-processing areas of your brain.

Step 2

I will show you how to integrate the pain competitor activities into your daily life. I also remind you of the environment you need to create to encourage new brain pathways to develop.

Step 3

The aim of this step is to provide a process for you to examine your own pain habits. I assist you to identify habits in your daily life, your physical and social environments, your thoughts and your emotional responses. Pain habits originally develop to help manage acute pain, but we look at them with fresh eyes to see if they are still your best possible response to pain.

Step 4

The goal of this step is for you to create a plan to develop new habits around pain. I show you a way to substitute new behaviours, thoughts and emotional responses to pain that will help you become happier and more productive.

Step 5

As we all know, pain is an ever-changing beastie. Some days, you have a spring in your step, whereas, on other days, you feel like you're walking through concrete. In Step 5, we consider how you can adapt your pain management strategies to respond to changing pain levels and everyday life commitments.

Step 6

This is where it all comes together. As we go through steps one to five, I will ask you to write things in the charts and tables in Step 6. This means you will have already completed Step Six, which is your personalised pain management program. Then, it is up to you to put it into practice.

If you have skipped the first section and 'cut to the chase' by opening the book here, there should be enough information in these steps for you to understand why we are doing what we are doing. I have started some steps with a quick refresher of key information. However, you might find that you need to dip back into earlier chapters to fill in the gaps.

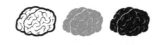

Step 1

Identifying pain competitors

Welcome to Step 1.

Think of this step as a new start for you in managing your pain.

A quick refresher

Here is a quick refresher of what you need to know to complete this step:

Acute pain can slide into chronic pain without you even realising it. Slowly, your life changes to accommodate pain. For some people, this change comes with fear, anger, sadness and/or despair.

Repeated pain messages of chronic pain have created and strengthened your brain's pain-processing pathways. In effect, your brain has 'learnt' to have a strong pain response.

Pain is processed in many areas throughout the brain. Our thoughts and actions can have an influence on eight of these areas, which are:

- prefrontal cortex

- anterior cingulate

- somatosensory areas

- posterior parietal lobe

- supplementary motor areas

- insula

- amygdala

- posterior cingulate.

These brain areas are also responsible for other processes, such as managing emotions or positioning the body.

You can think of the brain as a bunch of little factory. Each factory (brain area) makes a range of items, and some process pain as well. This ultimate multitasking ability of the brain is called 'dual processing'.

Over time, repeated pain messages mean that factories that have a side-line in processing pain begin to focus more on that and less on their other items, products or processes.

Engaging in specific activities, tasks or thoughts that require the pain-processing brain areas to use their other processes strengthens new pathways and weakens pain-processing pathways. This is called 'competitive processing'. Over time, competitive processing decreases pain.

I managed my pain by concentrating on four strategies to integrate competitive processing into my daily life. These strategies were related to:

- moving and being aware of my body

- being creative

- bombarding my senses

- connecting with others.

Now, let's take the first step

Step one in using your brain to manage pain is twofold. Firstly, we need to consider the emotions you have associated with pain and take those down. Secondly, it's time to identify the activities you could use to address the four strategies of moving and body awareness, being creative, bombarding the senses, and connecting with others.

I have included an optional third part of Step one, and that is to create your own tasks for pain competitors. To do this, I will show you how to analyse a task, and how to subsequently create or modify activities to enhance their competition to pain.

Taking the emotion down

It is not uncommon for people in chronic pain to be scared that something is seriously wrong with them. After all, pain is meant to be a warning signal, and fear is a natural reaction to that signal.

The brain itself is also contributing to our emotional responses, compounding our natural fear and sadness about pain. The extreme emotional responses you're feeling when you're in pain are partly from understandable sadness and fear, but also because the amygdala is overwhelmed with pain messages. As you may remember, the amygdala is responsible for managing emotions, particularly fear, and also is a brain area that processes pain. So, if the amygdala is busy with pain, our emotions are not managed as well as usual.

Interestingly however, there is some good evidence that people manage their pain better when they don't associate it with fear. If pain is seen as a simple sensation, albeit an unpleasant one, it is easier to manage than if the mind responds as if it is a warning signal.

When you are gripped by that familiar ache, or sharp hot stabbing pain (as it was in my case), there are some things you can do to take the emotion down:

Understand the processes

For many people, understanding the cause of their initial pain and how they have slid into a chronic pain lifestyle can go a long way to neutralise feelings about pain. For me, the fear was gone when the cause of my pain was identified, even though I knew that effective treatment was not likely. Once you know that you are not in danger, the fear and anxiety can start to disappear. However, even if you don't know the exact cause of your pain, understanding how the brain works in chronic pain still helps to decrease fear.

Remind your brain that the warning signal of pain is not needed

Although this sounds ridiculous, I found it helpful to remind my brain that I no longer needed it to alert me to pain. The danger had passed, so my brain could calm down. Sometimes I even went so far as to say this out loud (but not in public!).

Take control

Shift your focus from SEARCHING for a solution to CREATING a new solution. Try to think of your pain not as a danger signal, but as a challenge and an opportunity to rewire your brain. Being proactive in seeking your own solution (such as by reading this book) can make you feel in control again.

Identifying activities to compete with pain

Now it's time for you to begin to select pain-competing activities. I have put some suggestions under each strategy below to get you started. You can also skip back to Chapter 4 to remind yourself of the activities that worked for me. As you read through each strategy and their associated lists, make a note of any activities that appeal to you. If none of these jump out at you, I will talk you through how to create your own at the end of this step, ensuring that it will work as a pain competitor.

Body movement and awareness

I have a simple rule on choosing the right movement: find something you like to do. The goal is to move your body, at least 30 minutes a day, every day. You are not going to stick to that plan if you hate the movement you've chosen.

Enjoying what you do is also important in terms of neuroplastic change. To encourage your brain to change itself, you need to create a positive experience in which you can become immersed. That's not likely to happen if you're swearing under your breath for the whole session. Here is a list of potential activities you could do to force your brain's attention away from processing pain. Most of these activities involve moving, and all involve concentrating on your body's movement and responses. This list is just the beginning though. I'm sure you can think of more:

- Consciously and slowly relax all the muscles in your body. Relax your facial muscles and see if that sends a relaxation signal to the rest of the body.

- Remember what it was like to move without pain (mentally rehearse returning to this state).

- Break out that lycra and join an aerobics class (just a quick aside here: I recently found a YouTube hour-long wheelchair aerobics class from the late 1980s. It's exhausting and hilarious, with more than a whiff of lycra.)

- Pump some iron at the gym with strength training

- Find your inner peace with yoga or tai chi

- Create, grow and exercise at the same time with gardening

- Commune with nature by taking a hike

- Dance the night (and maybe your pain) away

- Pretend that your mother is about to drop in and vacuum until the carpet glows!

- Take a long, relaxing walk along the beach

Creativity

To compete with my pain, I used creativity and craft every day. But that might not be practical for you. Remember though, that many creative activities require similar neurological skills, so that means similar areas of the brain are being used for a range of different creative ideas. Feel free to mix and match your activities. Here are a few ideas to get you going.

- Get out your favourite cookbook and make a something that you've always wanted to cook but never had the occasion – battling pain is occasion enough to treat yourself.

- Get out the watercolours (or your kids' poster paints) and paint a picture.

- Write your autobiography, a family anecdote, or a Christmas letter (at any time of the year).

- Build something – upcycle a wood pallet into a chair, or a drink can into a candle holder. It doesn't matter how big or small.

- Take photos, concentrating on the set-up, the lighting, and all the other fancy things photographers look for. Then learn how to edit these shots on your computer.

- Plan your garden by choosing plants, then drawing them on a diagram of your yard.

- Use your creative thinking to complete word games and puzzles, such as Sudoku or jigsaws.

- Dance around the lounge room, in whatever style you like.

- Play a virtual world computer game and lose yourself in an alternative reality.

Bombarding your senses

Bombarding your senses to reduce pain can take on many forms. Here are some ideas:

Touch

- If you can't tolerate touch over painful areas, gently rub a nearby area, concentrating on how that feels on the skin.

- Concentrate on feeling different textures. Carry a small swatch of materials with different textures and concentrate on each one in turn.

- Brush your dry skin with a natural bristle brush each morning before your shower.

Concentrate on the invigorating scratchy-itchy feeling as you brush.

- Apply skin lotion after your shower, but don't just slap it on. Take your time and concentrate on the cool sensation.

- Find time to have a massage – professional or from a friend.

- Experiment with temperatures on painful areas – e.g. hot or cold packs.

- Rub your fingertips together, while putting all your concentration on that feeling.

- Lightly touch an area that hurts. Concentrate on the sensation and notice if touch changes the pain sensation in any way. Slowly increase pressure in your touch and note if that improves the pain.

- Rub different textures over your skin, such as soft fabrics, denim, and then a soft-bristled brush.

- Keep a smooth stone in your pocket, and when the pain strikes, slowly rub the stone, concentrating on its texture and coolness.

- Stand in a warm shower or wrap painful areas in a warm towel.

Taste

- Cook a comforting, aromatic meal and fill your kitchen with smells, in anticipation of great tastes.

- Find a food with a complex flavour, and take your time to savour it, trying to taste each element. My indulgence is dark chocolate with lime and sea salt. In fact, there is some in the fridge right now.

Smell

- Smell some peppermint oil. It's strong enough that you must pay attention to it, but it's also a pleasant aroma. Try a few drops on your shirt collar or use a 'migraine stick' containing peppermint oil on your temples.

- Sit in your garden or nearby park and concentrate on all the aromas you can smell. Try to name them, and spot where they are coming from.

Vision

Find visual activities that require focus and concentration.

- *Where's Wally* books. Maybe you might think this is a bit childish, but you could always do them with the kids.

- Jigsaws

- Word-finding puzzles

Hearing

- Music is the obvious choice here, but don't just listen to the music. REALLY listen to the music. What I mean is, listen to an intricate piece of music, and try to focus on one instrument, or one vocalist, at a time. Concentrate on hearing that one artist amongst all the other noises.

- Challenge yourself to sing along to a specific instrumental part of a piece of music you know well. (My chosen sing-along is to the bass line of 'Hungry like the wolf')

- Take a moment to sit still and listen to all the noises you can hear inside the room you are in, and then further afield. I can hear my dog snoring, my fridge rumbling, and the howling wind outside. Of course, until I was paying attention, my brain was ignoring those noises – except maybe for the snoring dog.

• Play an instrument or sing in a choir.

Connecting with others

If I were to ask to show me how you connect with other people, I suspect you would reach for your phone, not to call someone, but to open up social media. Am I right? Well, just hold on a minute before you do that.

I am not saying that social media is bad. It's a great way to stay in contact with people and to maintain long-distance friendships. But if social media becomes your only method of staying in touch, I think you would be out of touch pretty soon. Social media might then become a place where you feel jealous, angry and begin to think that life just isn't fair.

What I mean when I say connecting with others is just that. Building a connection, whether it be a minute- or life-long connection. You can even connect with someone you haven't met – such as by doing something for a charity organisation or for someone you will never meet. Here are some ideas for connecting with others:

- Provide help to someone else, whether that be by volunteering for a cause you believe in or helping family or friends.

- Engage in random acts of kindness, such as putting money in a stranger's parking meter, or paying for coffee for the person behind you at the drive-through.

- Help out at your local charity shop.

- Do something good for others, such as knitting hats for preemie babies.

- Get a pet and love it.

- Target the mirror neurones in your prefrontal cortex and insula to pick up on the positive emotions of others by watching a comedy movie.

- Laugh with others. It is always more fun than laughing alone, even if this means going to a funny movie alone (but with other people in the same cinema).

- Share a meal.

- Reminisce – call a friend who you haven't spoken to in a while.

- Think of one thing to do for the good of someone else and do it consciously each day.

It's your turn

Take time now to choose two or three activities from each strategy above, and write these down in Table 1 in Step 6.

If nothing on these lists takes your fancy, you might want to create your own activities that use pain competitors. I'll talk about how to do that now.

Analysing your own activity (optional)

If none of the activities listed above appeal to you, you might want to identify or create your own activity or adapt something that you already do to incorporate pain competitors. In that case, you need to undertake a task analysis to make sure you choose activities and tasks that compete with pain. A task analysis involves looking at an activity in detail and identifying what physical and mental skills are required. For our purposes, we are only interested in the skills that are used by the pain-processing areas of the brain.

To analyse a task, firstly, choose an activity (such as playing chess) and think about all the individual little tasks involved (for example, chess involves planning, picking up pieces, concentrating, etc). Then, return to the little brain factories in Chapter 3. Starting with the information on the pain competitor of higher thinking, identify which of the skills you use in doing these tasks. Move on to each competitor in turn. When you have gone through each competitor and selected a suitable activity (or three) that will compete with pain, add these to Step 6, in Table 1. Below, are a couple of examples.

Similar tasks, different pain competitors

I am going to walk you through two examples. Firstly, we will analyse two ways that people use to reflect on their life: journals and blogs. Then, we look at two ways of cooking dinner. Please note: I am not comparing each set of tasks to point out if one is better than the other, but to show you how similar activities involve different pain competitors.

Journaling: Reflecting on your day in a journal

Higher thinking skills required:

Memory – if you're going to write about your day, you need to remember what happened.

Planning – a journal entry can be structured and well-planned. Or, if you are a 'just get it on paper' kind of journal writer, planning can be at a minimum.

Decision making – you need to decide what goes in, and what is omitted from your reflection on the day.

Reasoning and problem solving – most people find that a journal is very useful to make sense of what has happened in their day, and to think through problems.

Concentration and focus – you might find that concentration and focus differ for every day in your journal. Some days might be difficult to write about, and you find yourself staring out into space. Whereas, an entry about another day may just flow.

Emotional skills required:

Emotional awareness – journaling usually involves some account of feelings for the day. You need to be aware of your emotions if you are to journal them.

Emotional responses and regulation – writing about your feelings can sometimes lead to relief, as you feel the day's emotions and let them go.

Pleasure – maybe, if you're writing about a good day.

Disgust – maybe, if the day hasn't gone so well.

Sensory information skills required:

Touch – holding the pen.

Visual perception – is the writing legible?

Body positioning and moving skills required:

Body positioning – positioning yourself in relation to the journal. Putting your hands and arms in the right place to write on the page.

Sensation of movement – moving the pen across the page.

Organising movement – moving the pen to write legibly.

Blogging: Creating a blog about your pain experience

Higher thinking skills required:

Memory – if you're going to write about your life, you need to remember what happened.

Autobiographical memory – backstory and context make a blog come alive.

Planning – a blog is likely to be more structured than a journal entry. It needs to conform to a style or structure so readers can make sense of it.

Decision making – you need to decide what goes in, and what is omitted from your story, after all, it is in the public arena.

Creativity – a blog is not just words. It is visual, stylistic, and some see it as a representation of themselves. All of that takes creativity, in that you are creating something that didn't exist before.

Concentration and focus – like journaling, you might find that concentration and focus differ for every blog post.

Emotional skills required:

Emotional awareness – for many, the emotional content of blogging is less than for journaling, but that depends on the content of your blog. In general, you need to be aware of your emotions if you are to blog about them.

Emotional responses and regulation – blogging about an experience can lead others with similar experiences to comment or make contact. You might have an emotional response to this contact, and you may need to regulate your response.

Pleasure – maybe, if you're blogging about a good experience.

Disgust – maybe, if your experience hasn't gone so well.

Empathy – by sharing your story, you are inviting others to empathise with you. Comments and contact from readers builds your connection with others.

Sensory information skills required:

Touch and pressure – pressing the keys on the keyboard effectively.

Visual perception and visuospatial cognition – does the blog page look as you want? Is everything in the right place?

Body positioning and moving skills required:

Body positioning – positioning yourself in relation to the computer. Reaching for the mouse and using the keyboard.

Sensation of movement – striking the keys on the keyboard or guiding the mouse with the trackpad.

Organising movement – coordinating your body to use both the keyboard and the mouse.

So, as you can see, both these tasks have similar-ish outcomes, but use different methods to allow someone to reflect on their daily life. The different methods mean that different pain competitors are used.

Here is another example where one task uses far more pain competitors than the other. Let's compare the activities of heating up dinner for one in the microwave and using the stove top to cook dinner for two.

Microwaving a dinner for one

Higher thinking skills required:

Planning – a small amount of planning in following the instructions and getting the required utensils, i.e. a fork to pierce the film.

Decision making – once again, a small amount of decision making required, but generally the instructions on the packet have made the decisions for you.

Visuospatial cognition – putting the frozen dinner in the microwave.

Emotional skills required:

Pleasure – maybe, but not likely with a frozen dinner.

Disgust – more likely.

Sensory information skills required:

Temperature detection – is the dinner still frozen in the middle?

Touch – carrying dinner to the table.

Visual perception – does the dinner look anything like the picture on the packet?

Auditory perception – the microwave ping.

Smell – this may or may not be pleasant.

Body positioning and moving skills required:

Body positioning – knowing where to place your arms to do the task.

Sensation of movement – moving to put the dinner in the microwave.

Location of external space – reaching for the microwave.

Organising movement – moving around the kitchen effectively.

Now, we will examine a second method of preparing dinner, in which a few crucial changes have greatly increased pain competitors.

Cooking dinner for two – on the stovetop, following a simple recipe

Higher thinking skills required:

Memory – where were you up to in the recipe again?

Autobiographical memory – almost certainly if you are cooking from granny's recipe of your favourite childhood meal.

Problem solving – not all recipes are easy!

Planning – following the recipe and getting the required utensils.

Decision making – you must decide what 'golden brown' means.

Creativity – using your cooking flair and magic.

Visuospatial cognition – chopping, stirring, plating up.

Emotional skills required:

Emotional memory – thinking about the other person for whom you are cooking dinner – not strictly necessary for the task, but you'll probably be doing it anyway.

Pleasure – hopefully.

Disgust – less likely.

Empathy – connecting with someone over a good meal – perfect.

Sensory information skills required:

Temperature detection – the essence of a warm dinner.

Touch – chopping, stirring, holding the pan.

Pressure – chopping.

Visual perception – does the dinner look anything like the picture in the recipe book?

Auditory perception – listening for the sizzle.

Smell – garlic and onion. Yum.

Sensual touch – maybe, if you cook like Nigella.

Emotional meaning to sensations – remember how much fun you had with granny when you cooked this meal when you were a kid?

Body positioning and moving skills required:

Body positioning – knowing where to place your arms to do the task.

Sensation of movement – chopping, stirring.

Location of external space – navigating around the kitchen.

Organising movement – chopping, stirring, holding the pan, standing by the hob, plating the dinner.

I hope you can see that 'cooking dinner' can use few or many pain competitors depending on how you do it. And this is the case for many types of activities, but you won't know which pain competitors you are using until you analyse the task.

It's your turn (optional)

To analyse your own activity, choose something you do every day. If you are stuck for ideas, maybe try a common activity such as playing a game on your phone.

Have a clear idea in your head of what that activity involves – what you do, where you do it, who you do it with.

Starting with the higher thinking pain competitor, identify the skills needed for that activity. Move onto the next competitor and continue until you have completed all the competitors' skills.

If you get stuck doing this, ask yourself the following two questions. Does your activity require many pain competitors? If not, how could you tweak it to require more?

In this Step, I provided many examples of activities that involve pain competitors. By using task analysis, you also have the flexibility to include and design your own activities. In the next step, we move on to creating those conditions in which your brain recognises as a time to change.

Step 2

Targeting neuroplasticity

In Step 1, you identified activities that would compete in brain areas that process pain – the pain competitors. By completing Step 2, you will develop strategies to make the most of these pain competitors to build new neural pathways and weaken the pain pathways.

Your brain has learnt to respond to pain ... a little too much. Now, we are going to unlearn that response by creating opportunities for competitive processing. We will be forcing the brain to focus on other processing task to minimises how much energy and space that brain area has left to focus on pain.

A quick refresher:

In the past, you possibly tried distraction as a way to forget about pain, and you might think that my suggestions for activities are simply a new take on that principle. But they're not.

Choosing specific activities for their ability to rewire your brain is different to choosing them because they entertain or distract you. We are not just taking your mind away from the pain. Competitive processing actually changes the structure of your mind.

Over time, doing activities that use pain competitors can decreases pain if neuroplasticity is switched on. But neuroplasticity only occurs in some circumstances. Not all new activities switch on neuroplasticity and bring about new pathways.

Neuroplastic changes occur when the brain determines that change or growth is in its best interest. Change happens when you are:

- working towards a meaningful task or goal

- concentrating on the task at hand and paying close attention to your actions

- faced with something new or unexpected.

Promoting neuroplasticity

Think back to the first time you sat behind the steering wheel of a car when you were learning to drive. Whether you were timid and scared or happy and confident, I bet you didn't have the radio blaring on day one. I suspect you hunched your shoulders, gripped the wheel until your knuckles went white, crossed your eyes in concentration, and stuck your tongue out so far that you were licking your own eyebrow. You might have even forgotten to breathe for a street or two. That, my friend, is the picture of absolute concentration. And in those (possibly) exhilarating moments, your brain began to lay down the foundation of new pathways for the action of driving a car.

Luckily, we don't need to recreate the pressure of that day to create new pain competitor pathways. However, we need to repeat the many positive aspects of the day your brain made new driving-the-car pathways, so we can encourage neuroplasticity.

Remember, the brain only changes in the right conditions – essentially when it is beneficial for growth or survival. For the strategies in this book to be effective, you need to create the right conditions for neuroplasticity. The following is what I did to promote neuroplasticity and control my pain.

Choose the right activity

The activities you select to combat pain need to involve at least one pain competitor. I described these competitors in Step 1 and provided quite a list of activities to choose from. By now, you should have chosen two or three activities that move your body, encourage you to be creative, bombard your senses, and help you connect with others.

You need to enjoy the activity. I can't say this enough! Chronic pain is already a chore; you don't need to add another burden to your life. Find an activity that makes you happy and immerse yourself in a new world. After all, pleasure is a pain competitor in itself, so the simple decision to choose an activity you enjoy goes a long way to challenging pain's processes.

To further enhance neuroplasticity, your chosen activities should be new to you, or at least, they must be things that you want to improve. The activities must involve learning or developing skills. For example, new learning might mean anything from picking up knitting needles for the first time, to extending yourself from basic knitting to a complicated, fancy knitting pattern.

Cut out the distractions

To encourage neuroplasticity, you really need to immerse yourself in a new non-pain lifestyle. And when I say to immerse yourself in a new world, I mean really be present. It's difficult to have full attention on a task at hand when the television is blaring or you are trying to multi-task.

Choose your activities carefully and then choose to concentrate on them. If that means finding a quiet space, or being alone, so be it. In saying that, on occasion, I would take my embroidery to a cafe (yes, I am unashamedly uncool), because, over time, I found that I could concentrate no matter how loud the conversation was at the next table (except if it was a bit saucy).

Practise and repeat

Learning any new skill requires practice. Each time you practise or repeat your selected activity, the pathways in your brain become stronger. Remember, our goal is for the new activity's pathways to become so strong that they take energy and space from the pain-processing pathways.

Ideally, you want to do at least one activity each day, for each of the strategies of body movement, creativity, bombarding the senses and connecting with others. If that seems like a large time commitment, think about how much time you have already wasted just being in pain. At times, I thought I was wasting my time too, but I battled on because the sense of doing something was better than sitting there in pain. Fitting these activities into my day was difficult at first, but slowly they became a habit. Here is how I found the time.

Body movement and awareness: I would start the day with a 30-minute yoga session. I logged in to YouTube in the spare room, and I would quietly yoga away in my pyjamas.

Creativity: Being creative has always had a place in my life. I'm not a big fan of television. I always have something half-finished somewhere in the spare room. As I mentioned earlier, if I was in too much pain to pick up some sewing or crochet (yes, I REALLY am that cool), I would do a jigsaw or colouring.

Bombarding the senses: This is the strategy that I found the hardest. When my pain was all encompassing, I couldn't stand noise or bright lights. So, I used mindfulness and meditation apps on my phone, and concentrated on the noise and feel of my breath. At times, that was all I could stand. However, at other times, I could quietly sit and savour the taste of a complex food (dark chocolate with lime and sea salt!!), or I could relax with a massage.

Connecting with others: At work, I made an effort to go and talk to my colleagues rather than send emails, when practical. After work, my friends routinely came around for dinner not knowing whether I would be cooking or whether we outsourced (i.e. take away delivery). They didn't mind because it was the company that we were all interested in, not necessarily the food. At these dinners, I banned friends from asking me about the pain. It wasn't because I was secretive, but it was because I wanted to take the focus away from the pain and back onto connection.

Practise with mental rehearsals

Have you ever wondered what the Olympic or Paralympic swimmer is doing on the blocks before the starter yells, 'get set'? They are mentally rehearsing their start, their strokes during the race, and their final tap on the wall – like they have done hundreds of times before. And why are they concentrating to do this and not just revelling in the atmosphere? It is because mentally rehearsing a skill strengthens pathways in your brain and improves your performance.

That is amazing! Quietening your mind and taking time to think about your chosen activity changes your brain! For our purposes, this means you can strengthen the pathways that involve your pain competitors even without lifting a finger. This is a boon on those days when the pain is so great that physical movement is the last thing you want to be doing.

So how do you mentally rehearse? Let's take tai chi as an example. (NB. to use this example, we need to pretend first that we are all familiar with tai chi and do it regularly.) So, here we go: Conjure a picture in your mind of your typical tai chi physical surroundings. In your picture, are you in a park? A recreation centre? A sunny room in your house? Then expand your thinking to the social environment in which you normally practise. Are you alone or can you feel the presence of other people?

Now, slowly, in your mind, go through every moment of your routine. Think about the position of your arms and legs, how your weight is distributed, when you inhale and exhale, the fluidity of your muscle movements. Are you imagining that you are moving slowly or quickly?

What information are you getting from your senses? What do you typically hear? see? smell? Are you standing on soft carpet? sand? a mat? Are you wearing shoes? Totally immerse yourself in your tai chi world.

Mental rehearsal practice can be done anywhere, at any time (except maybe when you are driving; your full attention is better directed to the road).

Practise even when you are in pain

For me, it was important to practise my competitive processing activities when I was actually in pain. It felt logical to battle pain, in hand to hand combat, during times when my brain's pain processing would be the most active. Actively fighting, whether it was by doing an activity or mentally rehearsing one, gave me a sense of control over my life. I felt like I was not at the mercy of pain and that it was not in charge of my life. By taking action, a sense of me, of my identity, returned.

But some of my activities were hard to do when I was in pain, so I had to develop a bigger plan. My strategy was to concentrate on a few activities that used similar pain competitors but had varying amounts of physical requirements. I alternated between these as required.

For example, when I was having a pain-free day, I would sit outside and do some embroidery. The pain competitors involved in this activity were mostly around higher thinking (such as planning, decision making, creativity), body movement (body positioning, organising movement) and information from the senses (visuospatial cognition, visual processing). But If I had some pain and felt a bit blaarrrgh (not a technical term but I'm sure you know what I mean), I would let myself retreat to the pain cave of the couch, but I would still do embroidery, not watch television (which was my usual pain cave activity).

If my pain was enough that I could not sit up, I would lie on my bed. Rather than sewing, I would use colouring in books. The set of pain competitors that are involved in colouring are similar to embroidery, but the bonus was that I was not that invested in the outcome of the task – I did not care if I coloured outside the lines, so it was perfect at that time.

If sitting up was too difficult because of pain, I used those same pain competitors to do a jigsaw on my iPad, while lying on my back. I picked difficult jigsaws, so I would need to concentrate. Sometimes, I would even challenge myself to find a set number of pieces in five minutes.

Finally, if there was just too much pain to even hold up an iPad, I mentally rehearsed sewing – once again, strengthening the pathways of those same pain competitors.

In Step 5, I will explain this further, and I will also give you some examples of activities that could go together.

It's your turn

Look at the conditions you need to create to promote neuroplasticity. Essentially, you need to challenge yourself to learn something new or get better at something you already do. If you have a serious go at the activity, try hard, repeat often, and concentrate on what you are doing, you have done your job.

Now in Table 2 in Step 6, write down how you will address each of these conditions for the activities you have chosen.

Next, in Step 3, we shift our focus a little from activities to habits.

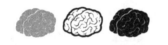

Step 3

Identifying pain habits

In Step 3, we continue to rewire the pathways inside your brain, and we move from pain competitors to pain habits. By completing this step, you will identify habits in your daily life, your physical and social environments, your thoughts and your emotional responses, which may inadvertently keep you in a pain lifestyle.

Remember, pain habits typically develop over time, with the sole purpose of helping you manage acute pain. However, they might have outstayed their welcome and now they restrict your life. Acting in habitual ways, whether that be habits of action, thought, or feelings, strengthens brain pathways that associate that habit routine with detection and response to pain. You need to break pain habits to reclaim your life.

In this step, we look at your habits with fresh eyes to see if they are still your best possible responses to pain. However, trying to examine an entire life in one go is difficult, so I am going to provide a few signposts to guide you to think about the following areas of pain habits:

- daily activities

- habitats

- thoughts

- emotions.

When you first examine your own pain habits, the most obvious component is usually the habit routine; the part that you can usually see or notice. For this reason, we will start by identifying your routines associated with pain. Then, we will work backwards to examine the cues of your habits, and then the rewards.

Identifying your habit routines

As discussed in Chapter 5, a habit routine is the behaviour, thought or emotion that comes about when your brain responds to a habit cue. It is usually obvious to you and is often the bit that others see too. For this reason, start with spotting your routines first, and ask your friends and family to help you to identify your habit routines around pain.

Here are a few questions to get you thinking about your own routines. These examples are common routines associated with chronic pain. Take note of the ones that relate to you and write the associated habit routine in the first column of Table 3 in Step 6. Then, write down any others that you think of that you do, think or feel.

Daily life routines – does your pain dictate how you spend your time?

- Do you spend more time looking at screens (tv, computer, phone) than you used to?

- Have you got an unfinished project or hobby in the cupboard that hasn't seen the light of day for a while?

- If you were a keen gardener before your pain, take a look outside now. What is the state of your garden today?

- Do you avoid physical exercise, even activities that will not increase your pain?

- When was the last time you met a friend for coffee?

- Have you started to drive for short distances – the distances you typically would walk before?

- If you were the cook in the household, have you continued to do that?

- Do you often get to the end of the day and feel like you have done nothing with your time?

Habitat routines – are you in a pain cave?

- Do you typically reach for a specific piece of clothing, such as an oversize jumper, when you are in pain? Is it something that you would not consider wearing out of the house?

- Do you sit in the same chair or lie on the same couch when you are in pain?

- Do you reach for the same comfort food or drink when you are in pain?

- Do you go outside less than you used to?

Thinking routines – are you struggling to imagine a life without pain?

- Do you find yourself thinking about your pain often? Are you ruminating on it?

- If the pain eases, do you think that it's only a matter of time before it will return?

Emotional routines – is your glass half empty, or even completely empty?

- Even if your doctor cannot find a reason for your pain, do you feel that there must be something seriously wrong?

- Are you angry at the medical profession for not being able to help?

- Are you scared to do physical activities because you think it will exacerbate your pain?

- Are you angry about all the things your pain forces you to miss out on?

- Does it make you sad to think of all the things you are unable to do because of the pain?

- Are you jealous of your friends who are not in pain and can do whatever they please?

- Do you feel like this situation will never end?

It's your turn

Think carefully about all areas that habits can change: daily life, habitat, thinking and emotions. Ask your family and friends what they think are your habit routines associated with pain and write these in the first column of Table 3 in Step 6.

Make sure you write them down. Seriously, don't move on to cues or rewards until you have written them down.

A wishy-washy habit identification will lead to a half-baked solution.

Just to get you started, I filled in a sample table for myself with the example from Chapter 6 where I unintentionally told myself I was in pain even when I was fine.

(If you skipped that bit of the book, here's a quick explanation: I had a pain habit that snuck under the radar for a long time, which I discovered after driving a friend home. When I got out of my car, sat in my wheelchair and reached over to take my keys out of the ignition, I said, 'Gee, my belly is sore'. It was not until she pointed out that I had just told her I was feeling good that day that I realised my belly was not sore at all. That statement was said out of habit.)

Table 3. Identifying pain habits

	ROUTINES	CUES	REWARDS
DAILY LIFE	Stating, 'Gee, my belly is sore' even when I was pain free.		
HABITAT			
THINKING			
EMOTIONS			

Identifying your cues

Cues are the catalysts that start a habit routine. They could even be described as a need that we want to fill, and the routine is the method by which we fill that need. Sometimes these needs are not obvious, and you might have to do some detective work.

As I described in Chapter 6, common cues come from the physical environment, the time of day, who you are with, and what happened just before. A good start when identifying cues of pain habits is to keep those common areas in mind.

Below, I have continued to fill in the table for my habit routine of telling myself I was in pain. I thought about when, where, and what was happening before, which gave me an idea of the cue for my habit routine. What I discovered was that it did not matter whether I was with people or alone, I said it out loud anyway. It happened at many locations and at any time of day. Over time, I figured out that the common thread was leaning forward to reach for something.

If you think about acute pain, that cue makes sense for me. In the beginning of my pain, my stomach hurt when I leant forward. But, over time, the pain wasn't always present, so I no longer needed to respond to that cue every time.

And here's the clincher about habits ... the cues sparks the routine even if that routine is no longer needed.

Table 3. Identifying pain habits

	ROUTINES	CUES	REWARDS
DAILY LIFE	Stating, 'Gee, my belly is sore' even when I was pain free.	Leaning forward to reach for something	
HABITAT			
THINKING			
EMOTIONS			

It's your turn

One at a time, consider each routine you have identified and written in Table 3 in Step 6. Think back to the last time that routine occurred and ask yourself these questions:

- Where were you at the time?

- What time of day was it?

- Who else was there?

- What were you doing?

- What happened just before?

Some cues will be obvious, but others can be a little tricky to decipher. You might need to wait until you are actually doing the habit routine, and then take a moment to answer those questions.

After a few times of examining a routine, you should find a common thread. The cue could be a physical task that exacerbates your pain, or even that you are bored and need company.

Fill in the next column in the table in Step 6 with your cue (just like I did in my example).

Identifying your reward

Rewards are powerful. Often, we go out of our way to seek them. Rewards of pain habits are no different. Obviously, the biggest reward sought by those of us with chronic pain is to be pain free, or at least for the pain to ease up a bit. However, sometimes, the goal, or reward, of our pain habits is a bit more concealed than simple pain relief.

The reward of retreating into a pain cave may be that you feel safe and in control. This is important if you are scared that your pain indicates that something is seriously wrong, and you feel that your life is spiralling out of control. It is not called a comfort zone for nothing!

But, it's possible for rewards to have a negative impact on your life. In the acute stages of pain, you might have developed habits that helped you cope at the time. However, in chronic pain, these habits might be holding you back. For example, you might be using a pain routine to fill in time. For example, if lying on the couch watching a movie has become the routine when you feel some pain coming on, you do not need to think of other ways to spend your time. You have created a habit that might ease some of your pain, but it won't help you interact with others, or to do things that are meaningful to you.

Here is my completed routine, cues and reward for my example pain habit. As you can see, the reward started as useful when I had acute pain, so it is logical that the habit became entrenched.

Table 3. Identifying pain habits

	ROUTINES	CUES	REWARDS
DAILY LIFE	Stating, 'Gee, my belly is sore' even when I was pain free.	Leaning forward to reach for something	Expresses how difficult I am finding daily activities and reminds me to be careful when I move.
HABITAT			
THINKING			
EMOTIONS			

It's your turn

After a bit of digging and examining your own pain routines and cues, you might begin to see a pattern of rewards that extend beyond simply easing the pain. You might find it helpful to identify what the goal of that habit was in acute pain because your brain probably still has that goal in mind.

For each habit routine that you identified, write down the reward that you were seeking (maybe subconsciously) in the final column of Table 3 in Step 6. I will show you how to keep these same rewards but shift your pain routines in the next step; for now, it is enough just to identify those rewards. Try to delve below the surface of 'pain relief'.

In Step 4, we will move on to reshaping your pain habits to reshape the way you manage pain.

Step 4

Replacing pain habits

In Step 4, we create a plan to develop new habits to replace those pain habits that you have held onto for too long.

By completing this step, you will learn how to substitute new behaviours, thoughts and emotional responses to pain that will help you become happier and more productive.

The goal of all habits is to get you to run on autopilot to save energy in your brain. Habits enable you to act, think or respond efficiently and effectively with tried and tested methods.

By their very nature, habits are notoriously difficult to break because you launch into habit routines without thinking about it. But, anyone who has successfully quit smoking or stopped chewing their nails will tell you that a habit can be broken. It is difficult, but it can be done.

Habit breaking

There is a 'shortcut' in breaking old habits. The key is to focus on changing only one bit of the habit loop. The most effective bit to change is the habit routine: that part of the habit loop that you see or notice. So, in effect, you will respond to the same cue, keep the same reward, but substitute a new routine for the old one. This is the technique I used to change my pain habits.

Returning to my example from the previous chapter, here is how I changed the routine of my pain habit:

When I leant forward to reach for something, I changed saying 'my belly hurts' (old routine) to 'Gee, that is a long way' (new routine) to express how difficult I was finding life and to protect myself by remembering to be careful when I moved. A simple change in wording gave me the same reward of reminding me to be careful but took away the reminder of pain.

Here are some other changes I made.

When my neuropathic pain was gripping my belly, lying flat would relieve some of the pain. Let's look at that habit through the eyes of the habit loop:

Old pain habit

The cue – neuropathic pain, horrible electric shocks of stomach pain, seven out of ten on the pain scale.

The habit routine – lying on my bed, with a cup of tea, watching telly.

The reward – hopefully, a decrease in pain intensity.

Although that habit relieved some of the pain, it also made me feel sad and isolated. I had retreated to the pain cave. But, by simply changing the habit routine, I took myself out of that cave. Here is the new habit I developed:

Replacement habit with brain-changing activities

The cue – neuropathic pain, horrible electric shocks of stomach pain, seven out of ten on the pain scale

The habit routine –

- On a nice day – lying on the grass in the nearby park, with a cup of tea, chatting to neighbours or reading a book (or just using the book as a social prop while I people-watched!).

- On a rainy day or if the pain was particularly bad – lying on the balcony chaise, with a cup of tea, sewing or colouring.

The reward – hopefully, a decrease in pain intensity, and it was usually successful.

Simply by changing the habit routine, I took myself out of the pain cave and employed one of my strategies: either connecting with others (in the park) or being creative (on the chaise). Having two options gave me a choice, but also allowed me to adapt to both the weather and how I felt on the day. I still acted on the same cue, and wanted the same reward, but I took control of the habit by changing the routine.

The brain-changing activities that you identified in Step 1 could be ideal to use as replacement habit routines. For example, let's pull apart another pain habit of mine, which was to use movies to distract myself from the pain.

Old pain habit

The cue – neuropathic pain, horrible electric shocks of stomach pain, eight out of ten on the pain scale

The habit routine – stop working on the computer and stream a movie instead.

The reward – hopefully, a decrease in pain intensity.

Replacement habit with brain-changing activities

The cue – neuropathic pain, horrible electric shocks of stomach pain, eight out of ten on the pain scale

The habit routine – stop working on the computer and play a Sudoku or brain training game instead.

The reward – hopefully, a decrease in pain intensity by using non-pain pathways in my prefrontal lobe (the higher thinking areas), and it was usually successful.

Changing your pain habits in the realms of daily life, habitat, thinking, and emotional responses will have varying requirements. For example, new routines for habits in daily life will take a different focus to new routines in the areas of thinking and emotions. A routine for daily life might be to focus on cooking a real dinner every night, when the routine for emotions might be to learn about the cause of chronic pain rather than feeling fearful of what might be happening.

Let's look at common habits in each realm and consider new activities that force pain competitors into action. I think that the combination of using pain competitors in your new habit routines gives you double the value from the one activity.

Daily life

Have you slowly but surely become a couch potato? If so, change your habit routine and engage pain competitors by doing some form of physical activity each day. It doesn't have to be going to the gym. You could dig in the garden, do some yoga, go for a walk.

Do you spend a lot of time in front of a screen – whether that be computer, television or tablet? Well, change your habit routine and engage pain competitors by taking up a creative hobby or learn to play an instrument.

Habitat

Check your posture when you're not experiencing pain. Are you still acting like it hurts? Change your habit routine and engage pain competitors by relaxing your facial muscles and let that feeling send a relaxation signal to the rest of your body. Consciously and slowly relax all the muscles in your body.

Do you feel like your life has lost the shine it once had? Change your habit routine and engage pain competitors by using aromas around the house that bring back memories of happier times. For example, pine oil might bring back memories of Christmas if you were lucky enough to have a fresh tree to decorate when you were a child. Reminisce with your family about pleasant experiences in the past.

When you are in pain, do you reach for the same snack as you retreat to your pain cave? Well, change your habit routine and engage pain competitors by treating yourself to something with complex flavours. Eat slowly, concentrating on identifying each flavour in turn. For me, my complex snack of choice is a piece of dark chocolate with lime and sea salt (I know I've said that already, but it's THAT good!)

Thinking

Have you been searching endlessly for a solution to your pain? It might be time to shift your focus to creating a solution. The first step is to understand the brain and body's responses to chronic pain. Change your habit routine and engage pain competitors by reinterpreting pain messages and renaming pain to 'nerve messages' or something of your choice. I found pain easier to cope with when I changed the name to 'pins and needles' (even though it felt more like 'knives and swords' at the time!)

Try to think of your pain not as a danger signal, but just as an anomaly of a nerve message or an overzealous brain loop. See an outbreak of pain as a challenge, and an opportunity to try reshaping your brain and take control.

Be firm in driving the action, knowing that the pain will try and stop you. Having a sense of control and purpose engages pain competitors.

Rather than trying to tune out when you are in pain, fully concentrate and explore what the pain really feels like. Where is it? What sensations do you feel? Is it hot? Cold? Constant or changing? In one place or moving? Thinking about pain in this way uses the pain competitors that interpret sensory information.

Do you think, 'There is no point? I can't do anything about the pain'? If so, acknowledge that your brain can relearn how it approaches pain, and you can direct that change. Counteract pain thinking.

Emotional responses

Understanding how your brain is reacting to chronic pain is the first step in helping the paint to abate. Once you know that you are not in danger, the fear and anxiety can start to disappear. For many people, the fear of further damage needs to be addressed to physically move forward. Fear stops people engaging in exercise and movement. Some researchers have pointed out that understanding physical mechanisms of pain can reduce fear.

If you think fear is holding you back, take moving slowly, but keep going. One of my favourite phrases is 'It doesn't matter how slowly you're going, you're still beating the person on the couch'.

Do you feel stuck in your own world, which centres on pain? Well, change your habit routines and engage pain competitors by finding something to do for the good of someone else, and do it consciously each day. If you can't think of anyone who needs your help, animals need help too. For example, maybe your neighbour would appreciate you giving their dog some company.

Has your life become a trudge through a list of chores? Is pleasure missing? Change your habit routine and engage pain competitors by doing at least one thing each day that brings you pleasure. It could be as simple as phoning a friend for a chat or drinking tea in the garden. Try to think of at least 20 things that bring you pleasure and work your way through the list.

It's your turn

The simplest way to change your pain habit, is to change the habit routine. Respond to the same cue and aim for the same goal or reward, but replace your old routine with a new one you have generated.

Choose one of your habit routines from Step 3, preferably the one that you think will be the easiest to replace. Refer to the reward column and try to identify a new habit routine that will give you that reward. Look at the lists above to start you off with generating ideas.

Write your plan, such as below, in Table 4 in Step 6.

When (cue) happens, I will (new routine) to (reward).

Concentrate on this habit for the next week or so. When you think that is under control, move on to another habit, and so on. You will find it is more motivating to start with the easier ones to change.

Next, in Step 5, we consider how you can adapt your pain management strategies to respond to changing pain levels and life commitments.

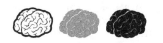

Step 5

Adapting to changing pain

By completing Step 5, you will learn how to adapt your pain management strategies to respond to changing pain levels and life commitments. Reclaiming your life from pain is not going to be a straightforward process. You will have good days and bad days. We want to shift the balance to more of the good and less of the bad, but this will only happen if you are consistent with fighting the pain habits and creating new brain pathways.

There are four key principles you will need to embrace:

- **combat pain daily**

- **fight when you are in pain**

- **value add to your activities**

- **avoid the 'boom or bust' downfall.**

I will explain each principle and give you an opportunity to apply each to your own situation.

Combat pain daily

Initially, don't be discouraged by little, or even no results. The way to stop persistent pain is to be equally as persistent in fighting it. Each time you use your pain plan, you are shifting the work of the 'brain factories', even if the pain does not shift in that moment.

Each time you force those brain factories to return to their main job and lessen their focus on the side job of processing pain, you weaken pain pathways.

There is no research yet as to how long an activity needs to be done to get the benefits of competitive processing. My method was to actively choose to be present for however long I could. I would aim for 30 minutes or so of concentrating just on the one pain competitive activity. Sometimes my attention would wander. In those moments, I knew I wasn't optimising conditions for neuroplasticity, so I would stop and try again later in the day. At other times, I got so lost in the activity, that time flew by, and before I knew it, hours had passed.

Like any new situation or skill, it was difficult in the beginning, but got easier over time.

It's your turn

- Go back to the list of possible activities you created in Step 1.

- Beside each one in Table 1, write whether it is an activity that you will do daily, every few days, weekly, monthly, on occasion or as a substitute for an existing pain habit.

- For each that you indicated you will do daily, write down the specifics of when and where you will do that activity. Try to aim for a minimum of 30 minutes for each of these daily activities.

- Do you need a reminder to do it? If so, could you link it to another daily activity? For example, if you plan to exercise and move your body 30 minutes a day, could you incorporate that in your commute to work, or by taking the kids to school.

Adapt to varying pain levels

In Step 2, I told you about how I could continue to challenge my pain-processing areas of the brain during varying amounts of pain. In short, I scaled up or scaled down the physical demands of activities but continued to challenge the same pain-processing part of my brain.

For me, the reason I was able to continue to fight pain was because I could keep my brain active while restricting how much my body needed to participate.

It's your turn

- To continue to combat pain even when you are hurting, go back to the activities you noted in Step 1.

- Try to think of a few similar activities that you like to do and that also challenge the same brain areas but that require different levels of physical activity.

- Nominate which you will do when in no pain, a bit of pain, and a lot of pain, and write those down in Table 5.

Value-add to your activities

Now you know the principles of competitive processing, and which pain competitors we are trying to use, it is obvious that you can target multiple competitors in the one activity. If you think about how, when, and where you do pain combating activities, you can easily target several 'brain factories' at once.

Let's take dancing as an example. Simply by tweaking something here and there, we can target various pain competitors.

	DANCING BY YOURSELF	DANCING WITH OTHERS	DANCING WITH OTHERS TO THE MUSIC FROM YOUR TEENAGE YEARS
Moving your body	✓	✓	✓
Responding to the sensory input of music	✓	✓	✓
Connecting with others		✓	✓
Reminiscing about the good times			✓

Another example could be cooking.

	Micro-waving a ready-made meal for yourself	Cooking a basic meal for yourself	Cooking an adventurous meal for yourself using a recipe	Cooking an adventurous meal for others using a recipe	Cooking a meal for others using a well-loved recipe from your well-loved grand-mother
Moving your body	✓	✓	✓	✓	✓
Responding to the sensory input of music		✓	✓	✓	✓
Being creatives		✓	✓	✓	✓
Concentrating			✓	✓	✓
Connecting with others				✓	✓
Reminiscing					✓

It's your turn

- Choose one activity from your list that you identified in Step 1.

- What pain competitor is it using?

- How could you add another?

- Write that down in Table 6.

Avoid the 'boom or bust' trap

As your pain decreases, you may be tempted to do more activities. On the rare occasions I was pain free, I tried to jam my entire life into a few hours – visiting as many people as I could, shopping, maybe even working! However, on those occasions, I pushed it too hard, I crashed and burned. Oftentimes, my recovery took a long time, longer than if I was sensible and paced myself.

I know you are tempted to do as I did, and that is to try and fit your whole life into those few sweet hours of pain-free living but try to be smarter than I was. Certainly, do more than what you do on your painful days, but remember, slowly does it. It is important to gently push yourself beyond what you thought were your limitations, but do this slowly and not all at once.

It's your turn

There isn't a 'your turn' for this bit. Just keep it in mind and be smarter than I was!

In Step 6, we will create your individual plan to break pain habits.

Step 6

Putting a plan into action

Step 6 is all about you. If you have been doing the 'it's your turn' activities as you go, you will have already completed your plan to rewire your brain's response to pain and break pain habits. If you wanted to read the book first, before completing the activities, great. Now go back and fill in the plan.

All of these worksheets are available as downloads from my website, www.lisachaffey.com.au.
You might find it easier to write these tables and ideas in a notebook rather than in this book (especially if you're reading the eBook). The notebook could double as a journal as you document how you are going in managing your pain. If you're not the journal type, no problem, just go ahead and fill in the plan on the downloadable forms.

Commit to your plan

All the lifestyle gurus out there agree that you're more likely to stick to a plan if you write it down. Writing a plan means that you have had to be specific about what you will do, how, when, and maybe even, with who. The more concrete an idea, the easier it is to follow.

However, there is another reason to write your plan down when you have chronic pain. Pain is all encompassing, and sometimes it is all you can think about. It makes you forgetful. So, writing down your plan of attack on pain reminds you of what you said you would do. All you need to do is follow the plan, not remember the theory.

The following tables and diagrams belong to Steps 1 to 5. I urge you to complete them all and follow your own plan to manage your pain habits.

Step 1. Identifying activities to compete with pain

Choose two or three activities from each strategy in Step 1, and write these down in Table 1.

Table 1

STRATEGY AREA	ACTIVITY	HOW OFTEN / WHEN (Come back to this column in Step 5)
Body movement and awareness	1. 2. 3.	
Creativity	1. 2. 3.	
Bombarding the senses	1. 2. 3.	
Connecting with others	1. 2. 3.	
Other activities you identified yourself (optional)	1. 2. 3.	

Step 2. Creating the right conditions for neuroplasticity

Answer the following questions about how you will create the right conditions for enhancing neuroplasticity for one of your pain-competing activities. Repeat this step for all the activities you identified in Step 1.

Table 2

ACTIVITY:	
Cutting out the distractions	
Where will you do the activity?	
Who else will be around?	
What time of the day will you do it?	
What distractions might be present?	
How will you deal with those distractions?	
Practising and repeating	
How can this activity become part of your daily life?	
Practising with mental rehearsals	
Where and when could you mentally rehearse it? (Hint: do you commute to work on the bus or train?)	
Practising even when you are in pain	
How could you adapt the physical requirements of the activity to reflect your pain levels?	

Step 3. Identifying pain habits

Remember, it is often easier to start by identifying your habit routine, and then move on to cues and rewards. Ask family and friends to help if you are having trouble on your own.

Fill in Table 3 with your pain habits.

Table 3

	ROUTINES	CUES	REWARDS
DAILY LIFE			
HABITAT			
THINKING			
EMOTIONS			

Step 4. Replacing pain habits

Complete the following sentence for all of the pain habits that you identified in Step 3

When (cue) happens, I will (new routine) to (reward)

Table 4

DAILY LIFE	When .... happens,
	(cue)
	I will ....
	(new routine)
	to ....
	(reward)
HABITAT	When .... happens,
	(cue)
	I will ....
	(new routine)
	to ....
	(reward)

THINKING	When .... happens,
	(cue)
	I will ....
	(new routine)
	to ....
	(reward)
EMOTIONS	When .... happens,
	(cue)
	I will ....
	(new routine)
	to ....
	(reward)

Step 5. Adapting as pain changes

Reclaiming your life from pain is not going to be a straightforward process. You will have good days and bad days. The key principles to adapt pain strategies to changing pain are: combat pain daily, fight when you are in pain, value-add to your activities, and avoid the 'boom or bust' downfall.

Combat pain daily

- Go back to the list of possible activities you created in Step 1.

- Beside each one, write whether it is an activity that you will do daily, every few days, weekly, monthly, on occasion or as a substitute for an existing pain habit.

- For each that you indicated you will do daily, write down the specifics of when and where you will do that activity. Try to aim for a minimum of 30 minutes for each of these daily activities.

- Do you need a reminder to do it? If so, could you link it to another daily activity?

Fight when you are in pain

To continue to combat pain even when you are hurting, go back to the activities you noted in Step 1.

Try to look for a few activities in that list that use similar pain competitors but require different levels of physical activity.

Nominate which you will do when in no pain, a bit of pain, and a lot of pain and write these in Table 5.

Table 5

NO PAIN	A BIT OF PAIN	A LOT OF PAIN

Table 6

Value add to your activities

Choose an activity from your Table 1.

....

What pain competitor is it using?

....

How could you add another?

....

Your plan

Congratulations!

You have just created your own map out of pain.

Table 1 lists the activities you have selected to compete with pain-processing pathways, and how often you will do each one.

Table 2 reminds you how you will create neuroplastic conditions while doing those activities.

Table 3 shows your current pain habits, and Table 4 clearly sets out your replacement habits.

Table 5 sets out your plan to continue to compete with pain processes while adapting to changing pain levels.

Table 6 gives you suggestions for adding pain competitors to an existing activity.

Pace yourself and change as much as you think will fit into your life. I tackled activities and habits all at once, but you might need to take your time adjusting your lifestyle. If you like, start with activities of competitive processing (Steps 1 and 2), and leave Steps 3 and 4 for a little while. Go at your own pace.

And that's it. Now you have the framework of a pain management plan.

And most importantly ...

Be relentless. Each time you do something that involves a pain competitor or changes a pain habit, you are helping. You are changing the pathways in your brain. It might take a while, but I am confident that you can rewire your brain's response to pain and reclaim your life.

Helpful sources of information

Brain changes and pain

Arden, J. B. (2010). *Rewire your brain: Think your way to a better life*, John Wiley & Sons.

Bushnell, M. C., et al. (2013). "Cognitive and emotional control of pain and its disruption in chronic pain." *Nature Reviews Neuroscience* 14(7): 502-511.

Butler, D. S. and G. L. Moseley (2013). *Explain Pain* 2nd Edn, Noigroup Publications.

Doidge, N. (2016). *The Brain's Way of Healing: remarkable discoveries and recoveries from the frontiers of neuroplasticity*, Penguin Books.

Hebb, D. O. (1949). *The Organization of Behaviour*, Wiley

Moskowitz, M. H. and M. D. Golden (2013). *Neuroplastic Transformation: Your brain on pain*, Neuroplastix.

Activities and pain

Booth, J., Moseley, G. L., Schiltenwolf, M., Cashin, A., Davies, M., & Hübscher, M. (2017). 'Exercise for chronic musculoskeletal pain: a biopsychosocial approach.' *Musculoskeletal care*, *15*(4), 413-421.

Busch AJ, Webber SC, Richards RS, Bidonde J, Schachter CL, Schafer LA, Danyliw A, Sawant A, Dal Bello-Haas V, Rader T, Overend TJ. 'Resistance exercise training for fibromyalgia.' *Cochrane Database of Systematic Reviews* 2013, Issue 12. Art. No.: CD010884.

Crawford, C., Lee, C., & Bingham, J. (2014). 'Sensory art therapies for the self-management of chronic pain symptoms.' *Pain Medicine*, 15(S1), S66-S75.

Kenny, D. T., & Faunce, G. (2004). 'The impact of group singing on mood, coping, and perceived pain in chronic pain patients attending a multidisciplinary pain clinic.' *Journal of music therapy*, 41(3), 241-258.

Kroll, H. R. (2015). 'Exercise therapy for chronic pain.' *Physical medicine and rehabilitation clinics of North America* 26(2): 263-281

Mitchell, L. A., MacDonald, R. A., Knussen, C., & Serpell, M. G. (2007). 'A survey investigation of the effects of music listening on chronic pain.' *Psychology of music*, 35(1), 37-57

Habits and pain

Dick, B.D., Rashiq, S., 2007. 'Disruption of attention and working memory traces in individuals with chronic pain.' *Anesth. Analg.* 104, 1223-1229.

Duhigg, C. (2012). *The power of habit: Why we do what we do in life and business*, London, Random House.

Kielhofner, G. (2008). *A model of human occupation: Theory and application*, Lippincott Williams & Wilkins.

Sjogren, P., Christrup, L.L., Petersen, M.A., Hojsted, J., 2005. 'Neuropsychological assessment of chronic non-malignant pain patients treated in a multidisciplinary pain centre.' *European Journal of Pain* 9, 453-462.

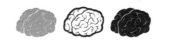

Acknowledgements

A simple, but heartfelt thankyou to my family and friends. I'm not going to single anyone out. You all know how you have helped, cajoled, encouraged catered for and heckled me (in a friendly manner, of course) to get around to writing this book.

CPSIA information can be obtained
at www.ICGtesting.com
Printed in the USA
BVHW041740140819
555664BV00061B/2440/P

9 780648 501008